YOUR CHILD'S RECOVERY

YOUR CHILD'S RECOVERY

A PARENT'S GUIDE FOR THE CHILD WITH A LIFE-THREATENING ILLNESS

BARBARA A. DAILEY

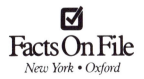

Facts On File
New York • Oxford

Your Child's Recovery: A Parent's Guide for the Child with a Life-Threatening Illness

Facts On File, Inc. Facts On File Limited
460 Park Avenue South Collins Street
New York NY 10016 Oxford OX4 1XJ
USA United Kingdom

Library of Congress Cataloging-in-Publication Data
Dailey, Barbara A.
    Your child's recovery : a parent's guide for
the child with a life-threatening illness
/ Barbara A. Dailey.
        p. cm.
Includes bibliographical references and index.
ISBN 0-8160-2347-6 (alk. paper)
    1. Critically ill children—Psychology. 2. Critically ill
children—Family relationships. 3. Stress (Psychology)
4. Adjustment (Psychology) I. Title.
RJ370.D35 1990
618.92'0001'9—dc20 90-13973
A British CIP catalogue record for this book is available from the British Library.

Facts On File books are available at special discounts when purchased in bulk quantities for businesses, associations, institutions or sales promotions. Please call our Special Sales Department in New York at 212/683-2244 (dial 800/322-8755 except in NY, AK or HI) or in Oxford at 865/728399.

Text design by Donna Sinisgalli
Jacket design by Levavi & Levavi
Composition by The Maple Vail Book Manufacturing Group
Manufactured by The Maple Vail Book Manufacturing Group
Printed in the United States of America

10 9 8 7 6 5 4 3 2 1

This book is printed on acid-free paper.

DEDICATION

To Shannon and Jessica, my true inspirations, may all of your dreams come to be.

To my father, William Moore, whose own life has been dedicated to assisting others, and who has shown me the gratification of giving rather than receiving.

To my mother, Kathryn Moore, who has sacrificed to provide me with insightful guidance and understanding of others.

To my brother, Bill Moore, whose support and encouragement have propelled my interests into reality.

To my grandmother, Kathleen Moore, who shares so much of her life and love to enrich the lives of many.

and especially . . .
To Stephen, for listening, understanding and loving, regardless.

CONTENTS

CONTENTS

6: Parenting

7: Siblings

8: Friends and Family

Appendix   143

Index   169

FOREWORD

One of the most formidable tasks that life can present is that of raising children. But among the many different life experiences that cause increased stress for a parent, few match the emotional anguish created by a child's illness. The anxiety and stress induced by a child's illness for family and friends is usually transient and easily reversible if the child recovers quickly and uneventfully. However, if the child develops complications of the acute illness or the illness itself is the first sign of a chronic or potentially life-threatening problem, then the situation is different. In all cases the parent assumes the role of the primary caregiver, coordinating advice from physicians and other health personnel with his or her own knowledge and experience. With close and effective communication, the parent can fulfill the role of the caregiver and markedly improve the outcome in a child with a life-threatening or chronic illness.

Thankfully, children have an amazing capacity to recover from potentially life-threatening illnesses with little residual problems. However, there are indications that chronic illness in children is becoming a more commonplace occurrence. The incidence of childhood cancer has been rising slowly but steadily since the 1950s. With improved treatments, more and more children survive for longer periods of time. It is estimated that by the year 2000, approximately one in a thousand adults will be a survivor of childhood cancer. Improved technology for neonatal care will continue to produce larger numbers of children surviving severe premature birth and the resultant complications. The expansion of organ donor banks and transplantation will lead to greater numbers of children surviving organ failure. Sadly, the explosion of AIDS in the adult population is likely to produce a new generation of children with congenitally acquired HIV-1 infection.

At the onset of a serious illness in a child, parents are faced with fear and uncertainty. During the initial diagnostic workup and initiation of treatment, parents and family members work through a number of emotions, which may include denial, guilt and anger. In particular, the near total loss of control over their day-to-day lives and uncertainty about their child's prognosis often overwhelms parents. The helplessness that parents experience over these issues can damage their faith and their identity as caregiver. Frequently, the child's illness can be the focal point for splitting a marriage or a family relationship previously weakened by other problems. In many instances there is ample staff and resources to assist these families. Approaches to dealing with families need to be individualized to the disease and to educating, supporting, counseling and helping parents resume their role as the primary caretakers and guardians of their child.

Frequently, after parents have had an opportunity to work through their initial shock they seek to learn more about the disease and what they can do to help their child. There are very few references available to parents that specifically address their role in helping the child with a chronic or life-threatening illness. In view of the impact of these illnesses on their families such a text as this one is vitally important for parents. The chapters in this book cover a wide range of problems parents are likely to face. The book also helps them come to grips with their role in their child's ongoing therapy. A parent serves as the crucial mediator through which any planned therapy must be implemented to reach a successful endpoint. More importantly, it gives parents an opportunity to resume the role for which they are best trained. Many parents try to take on too much responsibility for the medical aspects of relationships with their child, family members and members of the medical team. *Your Child's Recovery* provides a single up-to-date reference that gives the parent an opportunity to assume a vital role in his or her child's care that will improve the outcome, a reference that is unique and ideally suited to this important aspect.

Joseph M. Wiley, M.D.
Assistant Professor of Oncology and Pediatrics
The Johns Hopkins Medical University

PREFACE

When a child is diagnosed with a life-threatening illness, yet has the potential for recovery or extended life, the parent can have a significant role in supporting and guiding the child's understanding of the illness and normalizing his life as much as possible. This book attempts to discuss ways in which parents can participate in the recovery or adjustment of children diagnosed with serious illness at varying stages of development. While the possibility of death and the importance of helping the terminally ill child are acknowledged, the author's intent is to focus on the parent's role in promoting recovery or in normalizing the life of a child who has the chance for extended life. While various sections may appear more pertinent to some illnesses than to others, it is hoped that some aspects of the book will benefit all parents of children with serious illness.

Suggestions offered in this book are based on recommendations by professionals, parents, and people who have experienced a life-threatening illness, in addition to accepted research findings and the author's personal experiences. It is acknowledged that each child is unique, and parents should consult their child's health care team about any questions or concerns.

ACKNOWLEDGMENTS

I would like to acknowledge the following people for their support and willingness to share their expertise:

Dr. Donna Copeland
M.D. Anderson Cancer Center
University of Texas
Houston, Texas

Dr. Linda Dahlquist
Psychiatry and Behavioral
    Sciences
Ballor College of Medicine and
Texas Children's Hospital
Houston, Texas

Dr. Larrie W. Greenberg
Office of Medical Education
Children's Hospital,
National Medical Center
Washington, D.C.

Dr. Raymond Mulherm
Director, Division of Psychology
St. Jude's Children's Research
    Hospital
Memphis, Tennessee

Dr. Brian Corden
Pediatric Oncology
University of New Mexico
Albuquerque, New Mexico

Dr. Steven Goodman
Oncology and Biostatistics
Johns Hopkins University
Baltimore, Maryland

Dr. Roberta Babbitt
Behavior Analyst
Director of Outpatient Services
The Kennedy Institute for
    Handicapped Children
Baltimore, Maryland

Dr. Beryl Rosenstein
Director, Cystic Fibrosis Center
Johns Hopkins Hospital
Baltimore, Maryland

Dr. Joseph Wiley
Assistant Professor: Pediatric On-
cology
Johns Hopkins University
Baltimore, Maryland

The Johns Hopkins Childlife Department:
Jerianne Wilson, Director
Kathy Ziegler, Child Life Specialist
Joy Goldberger, Child Life Specialist
Bellinda Libbetta, Child Life Specialist

and especially,
Missy Deifer, Child Life Specialist

I would also like to extend my sincere appreciation to the Maryland Cystic Fibrosis Foundation, Maryland Easter Seal Society, Maryland Kidney Foundation, and the Association for Children's Health Care for prompt and courteous assistance with educational materials. In addition, a special thank you to Eileen Todd for her insights as a nurse and nanny to my own children.

1

THE PARENT'S
ROLE IN A CHILD'S
RECOVERY OR
ADJUSTMENT TO A
LIFE-THREATENING
ILLNESS

PARENTAL INVOLVEMENT

When a child is diagnosed with a life-threatening illness, parents may sometimes feel helpless as they see their child's life suddenly invaded by strangers, abrupt changes, and physical pain. For some families, their lives may quickly be thrust into a routine of medical procedures, diagnostic tests and treatment. Doctors and nurses may seem to be taking control of every aspect of the child's life. In other situations, many frustrating weeks, even months, may pass while the parent observes changes in the child's health. A doctor may examine the child and send him home, only to have the child return or be taken to another doctor. Finally a diagnosis is made, and the parent's fears or suspicions become undeniable fact.

This shocking experience is too complex and varied to say that any one parent or child should behave a particular way. We all have different backgrounds and experiences that affect our attitudes, including how we feel about illness, hospitals, life and death. A child's life has been physically, emotionally and psychologically uprooted. Lives have changed and a normal childhood seems like only a dream. Parents can see changes in their child's behavior as a result of hospitalization, medical treatments and fear of the unknown. In addition, the prospect of chronic care threatens to *alter* life for the entire family. At times, siblings may begin to feel frustrated and left-out, or burdened with added responsibilities. Spouses may quarrel or distance themselves from one another. Classmates and teachers can react in various ways when the child who is recently diagnosed returns to school. Through all of this, parents may begin to feel helpless and frustrated.

The family may feel overwhelmed, shocked, angry or perhaps numb as the child is thrust into this unknown world of medical technology. Today's health care experience can sometimes feel impersonal or rushed as hospital stays are shorter, medical staff are more highly trained but perhaps fewer in number, and treatments are more complex. Hospital routines, medical emergencies and financial concerns sometimes preempt support in the areas of parental, emotional, and behavioral issues associated with the illness and its treatment. While doctors, nurses, social workers, child life specialists, clergy members and other hospital personnel are available for guidance and support, counseling sessions are sometimes limited, and parents are unaware of what to ask before concerns arise. With technological advances and increasing rate of survival for many illnesses, new issues regarding emotional and developmental needs have now generated a new approach to helping families fight many illnesses and their effects on the developing child. So what can parents do to help their child and themselves through this painful and bewildering experience?

Over the past decade, parents have become more involved in determining some aspects of care. Continuing their parental role in the hospital, they assist with bathing, feeding and even at times giving medication. They assist in preparing their child for procedures, and they help educate him about the illness, treatments and procedures. Parents lend valuable information to the health team about the child's regular daily schedule, favorite activities, and ability to handle stressful situations. Now recognized as a significant support for the child, parents are participating more in the recovery process both in the hospital and when the child returns to home and to school.

A MESSAGE TO PARENTS

Only you as the parent can realize the emotional distress and unending challenges endured while supporting and loving a child with a life-threatening illness. Your experience is unique and it is not the author's intention to anticipate, compare or judge your actions as a parent. It is important to remember that while the parent's involvement can positively influence the recovery process, it does not determine eventual survival or death.

By understanding some of the beliefs and fears your child experiences during diagnosis and treatment, you will feel more comfortable and knowledgeable about supporting and guiding your child. Learning about the illness and its treatments *with* your child builds a binding and collaborative relationship that counteracts those frustrating feelings of fear, isolation and loss of control. A healthier recovery or adjustment to illness or injury involves open communication, ongoing support and the continuation of developmental growth. By supporting your child in these ways, you can help him to realize his strengths, abilities and true potential in life.

One thing to remember though is that you are human, not a super-being. You also need comfort, support and understanding. Accepting help from others is not a sign of weakness. When you feel things getting to you, it is important to take time for yourself. It may help to talk with others going through a similar experience. By seeking help for yourself, you will be emotionally and physically stronger to provide the much needed support for your child and family.

The only job more difficult than being a parent is being a parent of a seriously ill child. The normal woes of parent–child relationships acquire new direction, new emotion, and thus new challenges. While a successful recovery can never be assured, a supportive relationship can make the efforts rewarding for your child and memorable for you.

SO WHY THIS BOOK?

Thanks to advancing medical technology, many illnesses and injuries once considered fatal are now perhaps still life-threatening, but are more chronic in nature. The National Cancer Institute now considers several cancers, such as lymphoblastic leukemia, to be in this category. Many children with cystic fibrosis are now living into their mid to late twenties. Children with other diseases are now receiving new treatments or even transplants that provide greater opportunities for a more normal life.

This book was inspired by working with parents who sought more information about how illness affected their child's behavior and developmental growth. They were comforted to find that most new behaviors were normal responses to the new stresses placed upon their ill child. They were strengthened by learning what they could do to help their child and family through this difficult time.

This book serves as a reference for parents to browse through when they have taken a moment for themselves and want to learn new ways to help their child and family. It will also help parents realize they are not alone, and others are willing to help. Health professionals may find helpful suggestions for working with parents and families, and in turn may be able to help parents take part in their child's recovery process.

Though many suggestions are offered throughout the book, it is realized that real life experiences are almost never ideal. Sometimes the suggestions will help, other times they will not. They do, however, provide a starting point. It is also important to remember that there is no perfect parent (or perfect doctor or nurse for that matter), and occasionally individual values may differ. The purpose of the book is to provide suggestions with the understanding that people must work together, learn to communicate with one another, and put the ill or injured child's interests first. By promoting open communication that is comfortable for everyone affected by the child's misfortune, a more supportive environment is established. An understanding of the child's developmental level and potential fears or concerns also provides the foundation for

appropriate guidance and support to allow the child to feel more secure, and hopeful about the future. Parents are probably the strongest
influence on the child when he is ill, and they can serve a very important role in assisting him to cope.

2

TELLING YOUR CHILD ABOUT THE ILLNESS OR INJURY

WHY YOU SHOULD TELL YOUR CHILD
ABOUT THE ILLNESS

REASONS TO DISCUSS THE ILLNESS

We view children as carefree and fun-loving youngsters meeting the various challenges of growing up. It is normal for us to want to protect our own child from the pain, fear and confusion caused by serious illness. In the past, some believed that serious illness was a challenge too overwhelming for children and that they should not be told the prognosis or extent of disease or injury. This may have been based on the assumption that such discussions could be harmful to children emotionally and thus affect their chances for recovery. The belief that some illnesses would bring certain death helped to justify the idea that children would remain more peaceful and content not knowing what could happen. Today, advances in medicine have increased the chance of survival for many illnesses and have allowed for a reevaluation of what children should be told.

Research over the past decade has demonstrated that children need to feel secure about what is happening to them and that mutual trust among the child, parents and caregivers is of primary importance. These studies showed that fear of the unknown combined with an active imagination led many children to become stressed during illness, and their stress was compounded by a lack of trust of the people important to them.

Open communication during diagnosis, treatment and recovery helps your developing child to express beliefs, fears and misconceptions about illness. In addition, communication provides a strong emotional support for your child as well as your family. If your child is old enough to talk, talking about *what* he believes is happening and *why* helps you to understand his unique fears about the hospital, medical staff and procedures. Talking with your child, instead of *to* or *about* him, also may help to promote cooperation as he understands why all of these new experiences are happening. Children will usually feel more in control of the situation by being informed, and thus more willing to do as they are asked. It has been shown that educating the child about the illness may reduce stress-related complications (both physical and emotional), resulting in fewer visits to the doctor or hospital.

Some research has shown, however, that not all children want to know a lot of detail. In fact, some object to even viewing equipment that will be used in a procedure. Exposure to certain aspects of treatments or procedures may be too overwhelming or threatening, and the child's method of coping may simply be to say "I'd rather not know." Information should be offered, but parents and caregivers need to watch and listen to the child to see what he *wants to know*. Some children who initially deny the illness may eventually want to learn more about it. It does appear that most children prefer to know what is happening and why, but individual preferences should always be considered.

Your own child's perception of what is happening can strongly influence his emotional response to treatment. Imagine yourself in a brand new career, in a new office, with people telling you to do things without any explanation. If "Do as you are told!" were all that you heard, you would soon become frustrated, angry, or simply overpowered. A child in a strange hospital room, with little control over what people are doing to him, may feel the same way. Talking about what is happening is the first step toward being able to understand, cooperate and fight the feeling of being alone.

Lying (even lying with good intentions), avoiding discussions about the illness, or being distant only create more stress for children as they realize that they are seriously ill and their parents are very upset. Conversations held behind closed doors may be misinterpreted as discussions about bodily harm, tormenting death or even funeral arrangements. Sometimes, children may feel that they are not trusted, are too dumb to understand, or are unable to participate in the recovery process. A sharp and imaginative young mind can create many fantastic scenarios. Even a young child may establish an elaborate theory that the illness is punishment for kicking his sister in the knees last week. Unnecessary anxiety may develop if the child suspects that something is very wrong but the parents will not discuss this with him.

Children of different ages have various perceptions of illness and injuries. Preschool children often have strong imaginations, often termed "Magical thinking" and, as stated by R.E.K. Stein in *Caring for Children with Chronic Illness*, "From a child's perspective, nothing happens by chance . . ."[1] Preschoolers may feel that they have magical control over situations, or may fantasize about their bodies and what is happening to them. They often think that they did something to cause the illness. By explaining the particular disease in ways they can understand, parents can actually alleviate some of the anxiety and guilt that arises as a result of misconceptions about the illness and treatment.

School-age children and adolescents may confer with new friends during hospitalizations or clinic visits, and may compare diagnoses, treatments and particular medications. They can become engrossed in new relationships that offer frank discussions about bodies and illness. If they identify with the condition of another child, they may question their own treatment, or think that others are withholding information about the illness. Discussing the illness or injury can help reduce anxiety and increase feelings of self-control and thereby facilitate the child's return to school and normalize his life as much as possible. These are additional reasons to maintain an open channel for discussion of your child's specific illness or injury.

Regardless of your child's age, it is generally believed to be more beneficial for your child to be honest and straightforward about the illness and his feelings about it. The amount of information offered and the timing of the discussions will vary according to the complexity of the disease and treatment, the child's developmental level, and the willingness to listen.

"BEING STRONG" VERSUS SHOWING EMOTION

Families vary in the way they express their love for one another or express emotions. Some parents feel they must "be strong" for their child so that he will not become upset by seeing mommy or daddy crying. Other parents openly cry, scream or demonstrate anger toward health professionals when the child is first diagnosed. No one can tell you what is right or wrong for your family, or how to share your feelings, but the following should be considered.

- ◆ Does your child ever see you cry at home? If so, does he react? Does he become upset or scared, or is he empathetic?
- ◆ If your child sees that it is okay to cry, he can avoid the stress of holding back a child's natural response to fear—crying.
- ◆ Crying can be an appropriate outlet of emotion that shows concern and love for your child and assists with coping.
- ◆ Openly discussing feelings provides a secure and loving relationship with less fear of doing something wrong or "abnormal."

It can be helpful, then, to acknowledge your feelings and your need to cry. Then after a few moments, when crying has appeared to relieve some tension, direct the child's attention to something else. Parents who become overly affectionate in the hospital, compared to when they are at home, may lead the child to believe that he is dying. Emotions communicate a depth of feeling but at times can be misunderstood. If the diagnosis and prognosis are openly discussed, the parent's affection may be seen as support rather than "babying" or hiding the truth. Each family, however, expresses emotion in different ways, and only parents can decide how comfortable they are showing their emotions in front of their ill child.

COMMUNICATING WITHOUT TALKING

Our behavior reveals much about how we feel. We tend to forget how attentive and sensitive children are to our nonverbal language. We may say one thing, but our body language often reveals our true thoughts. Eyes that have become red and swollen from crying *are* noticed. Tapping fingers, nervous pacing, arguments between you and your partner, or "staring" at your child all reveal that you are tense or worried. It is very difficult for you as a parent not to show concern. Being more conscious of your actions and behavior, however, can help provide a more comforting atmosphere. Supportive behavior may include holding hands or cuddling to provide comfort, using eye contact to show that you are listening and interested when someone else is talking and smiling to show you are glad to be with someone.

Additional information about communicating with your child through play is provided in Chapter 4.

HOW DO YOU KNOW WHAT TO SAY?

Each child develops at his own pace, reaching different physical, cognitive and emotional milestones when he is ready. The manner in which a child will be told about an illness or injury will often depend on his age, developmental level and previous hospital experiences. In most cases the physician begins the discussion so that he can answer specific medical questions. Parents, if they are present, can help the child understand the explanations. The parent is never expected to be the one to explain the illness, but he may participate if he feels comfortable. Some parents prefer to talk with the child in private, without the presence of medical staff. This is a personal choice, and parents can discuss this with the physician, making sure they feel comfortable with the information they will tell the child. Parents can best gauge the child's moods and temperament. If possible, parents should choose a quiet time when there are few chances of interruptions (although this may be difficult during early diagnosis, when many diagnostic procedures are necessary).

In general, deciding what to tell your child may actually be determined by him. It has been suggested to first let your child express his own feelings and ask questions that are important to him. Supporting your child in this way shows that you are listening and are willing to share his fears. Acting as if nothing is wrong only denies personal feelings and the chance to express them. You can also paraphrase the physician's discussion of the diagnosis, medications and treatments. For example, you might say "The doctor says you are very sick and you need special care and medicine here in the hospital. Just like the doctor, Mommy and Daddy want you to feel better, so you'll be staying here for a little while."

The child's developmental level determines how well he is able to express himself or indicate what he does not understand. Some preschoolers or young school-aged children may demonstrate, by playing with a doll, that they are afraid a needle will drain all of their blood, as a vampire would. Some children may believe that the illness is a punishment for being bad. Other children fear that family members will "catch" their illness. In regard to therapy, children can become confused if some treatments are repeated or changed during the course of the disease, and discussions may need to be repeated or updated to explain decisions regarding their care. For example, if a child is treated with intravenous antibiotics, it is necessary to explain any adjustments that might need to be made to the medication or the dosage. If the first medication was not effective, he may fear that no medication will work. As a child matures, he may be able to understand more detailed information about his condition. Many believe a positive adjustment to the disease is correlated to early knowledge about the illness. As discussed later, however, normal aspects of your child's life should also be frequent topics of discussion to provide a break from "medical talk."

SHOULD DEATH BE MENTIONED?

For life-threatening illness, some believe that at diagnosis, or shortly thereafter, the word "death" should be mentioned so that it can be dealt with openly. This is often the most difficult aspect of the diagnosis for parents to discuss with their child. You may discuss the aspect of death with your child's physician to determine if and when it is appropriate to have this conversation with your child. Some physicians do not discuss death, in an effort to concentrate therapy on recovery and treatment. If you or your child are concerned about the possibility of death, though, talk about it. It is important to discuss *any* questions you have to promote a better understanding of your child's disease or injury and its prognosis. Some researchers feel that children over the age of 10 are more apt than younger children to be concerned about the aspect of death. Others, however, believe that even young children need the opportunity to express their fears and concepts of death, especially when death is a distinct possibility.

Children of various ages have different concepts of death. Some feel that preschoolers may confuse death with separation or sleep, or that it may be viewed as a violent retaliation for bad behavior. School-age children begin to understand that death is real and inevitable and that it is irreversible. Your child's experiences with the death of pets or family members can also affect his understanding of the finality of death. If death is discussed, it should not be equated with sleep. Confusion of the two can lead to fears of sleeping or having an operation.

According to the National Institutes of Health booklet "Talking With Your Child About Cancer," some parents feel better about rehearsing a discussion about death or any other aspect of the illness before sitting down with their child. There is no need to feel embarrassed about wanting to do this as a way to better prepare yourself. It is generally advised that parents be present when the child is told about the illness or possibility of death. Some adolescents, however, approach their physicians about the subject on their own, often in an attempt to "protect" their parents.

It is best to discuss these apprehensions and concerns with your child's physician, who is available for support as well as information. More information concerning fears about death are detailed in Chapter 4.

SUGGESTIONS FOR WHAT TO SAY BASED ON YOUR CHILD'S AGE

Once again, there are many reasons for parents to discuss the diagnosis of an illness with their child. One thing to remember is that the child will usually ask the questions that are important to him. If your child does not ask, you might begin a conversation by saying, "Is there anything else you would like to know about your illness?" Through discussion and play, you and the health professionals should be able to help your child to express his greatest concerns. The following are guidelines to help you understand what you or the doctor might say based on your child's age and developmental level.

ONE AND TWO YEARS OF AGE

Children under two years of age are learning about their bodies and the world around them. The parent is the main filter between the child and harmful things. Aware of sudden changes, a new environment, and painful experiences, a child in this age group has little understanding about illness. He knows only that it doesn't feel right and he wants to be home. It is important for parents to accept these feelings, and, as difficult as it seems, to simply comfort the child.

The illness is generally explained as "being sick," avoiding complex discussions that can create confusion or unnecessary fear. Children aged one to two have difficulty understanding how several events can be related, and thus they may not understand how the illness is affecting the body or why medicine is necessary. Simply explain that he needs to be in the hospital for extra special care that will help him to get better. Perhaps remind your child that you want to be home with him, but you want even more for him to feel good again. Emphasizing that you asked the doctor to help him get better might promote more trust in medical personnel. Explanations about procedures and treatments are usually offered by the medical staff just before they occur. Explanations made to a child long in advance of a procedure will only increase his anxiety and confusion when the event does not occur right away. When your child is told about a procedure, he will no doubt protest and become upset. Simply provide support to cope.

It is often difficult for parents to know that their young child is going through painful procedures during diagnosis and treatment. Repeated explanations that this is necessary for him to get well may seem to go unheard. Remaining calm and supportive can convey your trust in hospital personnel. Even though your child may be very frightened, this display of trust may help him to get through the procedure. Simply support your child before and after the procedure with love and affection. Playing or offering distraction after the procedure can ease the child back into feeling more secure and also offer an opportunity to vent any frustrations. Rewarding your child with favorite treats may also offer incentive to get through this tough time. Additional suggestions are provided in Chapter 3.

TWO TO SIX YEARS OF AGE

Children can usually identify visible parts of the body by the time they are four years old, but they might not understand how internal organs work or how illness can affect different parts of the body at the same time. Children aged two to six usually look at illness in terms of "cause and effect." The illness may be thought of as a bad cold caught as a result of not wearing a coat or from not eating the right foods.

One way to explain certain illnesses is to describe "bad" cells attacking "good" cells in the body. A child can understand that taking medicine will help the "good" cells to beat the "bad" cells. It should be emphasized that the bad cells were not a result of anything the child did. Another general explanation may be to say that the heart, lungs or kidneys have sick cells that need help to work right. Depending on the child's developmental age, more detailed explanations may include how procedures help the doctors to find where the "bad" or "sick" cells are and that the procedures will help the doctor to know what medicine is needed.

If transplantation is necessary, further explanation about why the child will get a new "healthy" organ to make him feel better may be offered. These children may need extra support in coping with the prospect of "losing" a part of their body, but they may be reassured that it will be replaced. Your physician may be able to offer pamphlets or coloring books for your child's specific illness to help him to understand. The hospital may have a special doll that can be used to explain body organs or procedures. Some organizations offer literature or videotapes specifically for children. The medical staff or social worker may help you to call or write to the proper organization for this material. A list of organizations is provided in Appendix A.

Children in this age group often have what is termed "magical thinking." Their vivid imaginations and creative minds often have difficulty separating fantasy from reality. They may imagine illness as a monster invading the body, or as an evil spell cast upon them. Medicine may be viewed as a special potion that will rid the disease as soon as they have had the first dose. Ongoing treatment may therefore be confusing. At this age children are also very self-centered and more sensitive to what is right or wrong. They want to please mom or dad by doing things the "right" way. A child two to six years old may feel the illness or injury is a punishment, or may fear that he did something to cause it. Talking and playing with your child helps him to express his beliefs and is also important for encouraging open discussion in the future.

Children in this age group may actively protest medicine or procedures, and repeated explanations may seem to be unheard or misunderstood. Preschoolers often express their growing independence and they strongly believe what they are thinking. They also may be troubled by fears of how their bodies will be harmed by medical procedures. The parent can help by patiently explaining the illness and procedures at a level the child can understand. Play therapy, which is often available on a hospital's pediatric floor, also helps children to act out their active imaginations and express their normal fears of being harmed. Again, the medical personnel are available to advise you on what to say. Coloring books focusing on hospitalization or the particular illness help to promote a better understanding by providing visual information and the opportunity to ask more questions.

SIX TO NINE YEARS OF AGE

Children aged six to nine are better able to understand additional aspects of an illness. Some conversations may be based on a general discussion of how the illness is affecting the body and how medicines or certain procedures help to fight the disease and protect the body. Some specialists feel that "children of this age can utilize information about causation, diagnosis, and treatment to reduce anxiety."[2] When your physician explains the diagnosis, medications or procedures, listen to what he tells your child and what questions your child has. If the physician does not speak directly to your child, do not be afraid to ask that he do so. This is particularly important if you are not yet comfortable with the medical terms or if you do not fully understand the illness or treatments. A family conference with the medical staff often helps communicate simple, honest and specific information important to your child. If procedures or treatments are to be continued at home, written instructions and a telephone number of someone to contact for questions or concerns can be invaluable.

Depending on your child's previous life experiences and exposure to illness, the name of the illness may or may not be associated with death. If a family member has died or become very ill from the same disease, it would be natural for your child to assume the same may happen to him. You may also be inclined to associate the illness with your own experiences with friends or family. It is also important to note if your child associates his disease with a different one he has heard about. Explaining how the illness is different can help to minimize confusion. On the other hand, if your child has often recovered from illnesses without difficulty, he may expect this illness to clear up as quickly as any "bad cold." Once again, discussion about your child's perception of the illness will help you and the medical personnel to decide what to tell him. It is recommended throughout the literature that you be truthful and be as optimistic as is appropriate.

NINE TO TWELVE YEARS OF AGE

Children at this age are able to understand illness as a progression through several stages. Brief discussions on how affected organs or body parts function may help you and your child to understand the disease process. Explaining that different cells work together may help your child to understand why a "sick cell" may affect the work of healthy cells. Some children ask for more detailed explanations. Let your child lead the conversation when he expresses interest. Your physician may help you determine if it would be beneficial to explain in more detail.

When the doctor does explain the disease to you and your child, ask for booklets that you can review together. Illustrated booklets offer valuable information, and looking at pictures may help you to understand bodily functions and the particular illness. Specific medical questions will of course be directed to the doctor, but you can help your child by learning alongside him. Your child's interpretation of information may differ from yours, and reviewing it together provides the opportunity to clarify misconceptions or the need for more information. If you do not know an answer, just say so. Writing down your questions will help you remember what to ask the next time you see the doctor. This will also show your child that it is okay to ask questions without feeling ashamed.

TWELVE YEARS AND OLDER

The older child is better able to grasp detailed explanations of bodily processes and how they work together. Once again, reviewing information together will help you both to understand your teenager's illness. Learning about specific body cells or how organs function together can help you to understand how treatment will help fight the disease or heal an injury.

The adolescent benefits from direct conversations with the physician and medical staff. By taking responsibility for his own education about the disease, he can establish some sense of control. If at first your teenager prefers to have you ask questions about medications or procedures, you can do so until he is ready to participate. Your encouragement and guidance may be necessary at times to facilitate cooperation or prepare your adolescent for necessary treatments. Continue to allow your teenager the opportunity to ask questions.

THE IMPORTANCE OF COMMUNICATION

An open communication network between the medical staff, the family and the seriously ill child, helps the child to accept his illness and deal with it appropriately. It has been shown that enabling a child to discuss the illness not only reduces feelings of isolation but also helps him realize that the illness is not so horrible that no one will talk about it.

Open communication also gives the opportunity for fun-filled discussions about happy things, especially activities the family looks forward to, and helps to maintain the family's morale. Everyone needs to forget about the illness for a time. Talking about different types of feelings can relieve the child or family members from the burden of trying to hold back emotions, and gives everyone the chance to have his feelings acknowledged and accepted.

FOR YOUR CHILD

To help your child deal with illness, encourage him to tell others how he is feeling before, during and after stressful times. It is normal to be angry, scared and frustrated. Some children, however—especially younger ones—find it difficult to express in words exactly what they are feeling. Instead, these feelings can be communicated through actions, and they will vary from child to child.

In times of stress, it is not unusual for parents to observe frequent crying or whining, yelling, acting out, biting nails, fighting with siblings, clinginess, or periods of silence. Some children may relieve tension through more aggressive play, such as banging toys loudly, hitting dolls, or punching or kicking balls. Children who are bedridden or are unable to use an arm or leg can become frustrated simply by not being able to express themselves physically in a way they are used to. They may become uncooperative, start to throw things, refuse to talk or try to ignore certain people.

Some parents become upset or worried when they see this behavior. It is helpful to realize, however, that this release of tensions is healthy, as long as the activity is not dangerous. Helping the child to channel this energy appropriately will help him to cope. Therapeutic play and other suggestions are covered in Chapter 4.

It helps support your child if you show respect for these feelings. If he cries, offer tissues. If he verbally lashes out or has a temper tantrum, tell him it is okay to be angry, but guide the anger to a more appropriate activity (for example, offer to hold a pillow or punching bag for him to punch). Then when things are calm, give him a big hug.

Subtle ways to encourage communication may include drawing pictures or taking a walk together. Talk occasionally about new friends or a favorite doctor or nurse. Before any new procedure or operation takes place, ask your child if he has any questions for you or the doctor. In this way you can discuss new concerns as they arise.

There may be times when your child will not want to talk. Respect this as well. If your child wishes to be alone, and you feel it is appropriate, offer to leave for a little while, emphasizing when you will return.

When you do wish to speak with your child, especially about the illness, it is important not to present too much information at one time. You can avoid confusion by listening to your child's questions and answering only what he wants to know.

Finding the right words can be difficult for the parent. When preparing the child for specific medical procedures, it helps to explain in simple terms what will happen and why, and how the child will feel during the procedure, as categorized below: For example, you can begin by describing the sensory experience including what he will see, hear, and smell, as well as what he will feel. If there will be any discomfort, discuss ways in which he can distract himself, such as by counting or imagining his favorite things. It may also be helpful to let him know if there are any ways he can participate in the procedure such as applying a bandage. Finally, let him know where you will be.

Remembering that some words sound more harsh or negative than others might help to guide the conversation. Researchers at Phoenix Children's Hospital have suggested that some terms be used instead of others to avoid confusion and minimize anxiety. A list of terms, assembled by the Johns Hopkins Child Life Department based on this research in Phoenix, follows:

WORDS TO AVOID WHEN POSSIBLE	SUGGESTED WORDS OR PHRASES
Hurt	Uncomfortable, different
	Pinch, sting, "ouie"
	Sore, ache
Shot, injection, poke	Needle
Stretcher ("stretch her")	Special bed on wheels
Put to sleep, anesthesia	Special sleep, help to sleep
Cut open, incision, make a hole	Small opening
Dye ("die")	Medicine to help the Dr. see
X ray, CT scan, MRI	Picture, special camera
ICU ("I see you")	Intensive care, special care
OR table (for operating room)	Bed
Funny smell/taste (too comical)	Different, unusual smell/taste

Because children perceive pain differently and the degree of pain can vary with the procedure, it may be advisable *not* to say "this will hurt," even when you want to be honest. You would be just as honest to tell your child that you are not sure how the procedure will feel, but that other people have said it feels like pressure, tingling, pulling, a pinch, a warm/hot feeling, a mosquito bite, a kitty scratch, etc. If your child absolutely insists on knowing whether or not it will hurt, however, do not say "no" if it will. It is important to maintain trust at such a confusing time. When you want to emphasize that he will *not* feel pain from a procedure such as an X ray, you can say "You won't feel anything unusual or different," rather than mentioning the word "hurt" or "pain."

Children can ask very detailed questions. You may sometimes feel like a walking encyclopedia or a broken record. Children may ask the same question over and over again to assure themselves they understand what they are hearing and know what to expect. They may sometimes even ask questions that you never thought of, and you may not have an answer. Once again, do not be afraid to ask assistance from medical personnel in the hospital. Different people offer explanations in different ways, and perhaps one person will define things in a way you both can understand better. This is a confusing time and you must not hesitate to ask the same question until you understand the answer. The stress of illness and a new environment often make you and your child nervous and in turn can easily make you forget all the new information you just learned.

FOR THE MEDICAL STAFF

Some parents begin to realize that the way they interact with the medical staff may influence their child's willingness to talk about various aspects of the illness, treatments or hospital procedures. If you communicate openly and in a matter-of-fact tone with professionals, your child is more apt to feel secure about what he is being told. Screaming at the medical team (which can happen as a result of stress or fear) can be stressful for your child and can alienate you from the staff. Additional information about understanding your own emotions and actions is provided in Chapter 6.

Researchers have found that in early diagnosis, the following concerns are most frequently discussed between physicians and parents: diagnosis, prognosis, disease process, additional tests necessary or recommended, immediate plan of care, and the physician's availability. These areas are discussed at different stages, depending on the child's illness and health status, the parents' or child's need for information, and the urgency of care. Some physicians may withhold information in an effort not to overwhelm the family. As a parent, however, you have every right to ask about what concerns you or your child.

Parents and medical staff may occasionally disagree on one or more aspects of treatment or care. One reason may simply be differences in experiences. Doctors, nurses, social workers and other health care workers develop attitudes, beliefs and knowledge not only from their educational and professional training, but from personal experience with illness as well. Parents, on the other hand, have their own values and experiences with the child and may have had exposure to different methods of health care in the past. While it is expected that parents nor staff will fully articulate their personal concerns or views, some researchers feel that "most parents are still intimidated by medical authority and are reluctant to confront physicians directly with their concerns."[3]

You are the best advocate for your child, and you should not be afraid or ashamed to share your thoughts. As previously mentioned, the way you convey your thoughts will effect how and what changes will be made. It has also been suggested that you "discuss any disagreements or dissatisfactions you have about the child's care with the medical team. But avoid airing your grievances in front of the sick child."[4] Establishing trust in professionals is necessary to continue the treatment relationship in an effective manner, permitting mutual participation of child and family and focusing on coping rather than on negative aspects of hospitalization. Additional information about dealing with health professionals is available in Chapter 6.

Your relationship with the medical staff may have some impact on your child's perception of the hospital environment and his experience there. This includes how you reinforce the necessity of prescribed medicines and procedures and your encouragement of the child's cooperation and participation in the treatment process.

It has also been suggested that parents who need to leave the child for a time should speak with the nurse in front of the child just before leaving. This conveys trust to the child and also lets him know that you feel comfortable about leaving him in someone else's care. The child may still protest about the parent leaving, but will feel more secure about the person who will respond to his needs.

While all parties must participate to a certain degree in decisions about medical treatment, sometimes parents or their child may feel overwhelmed by their participation in care. As one patient with cystic fibrosis points out, the relationship between patients and medical staff requires the balancing of the need for independence and responsibility with the need for rest and to be cared for.[5] This can also apply to parents, who often want to participate and help during recovery but also need time to sit back and simply enjoy being with the child.

Parents and children may also be overwhelmed by a physician's or nurse's use of excessive medical terminology. Medical staff sometimes forget they are using words that are not familiar to the parent or child and will forget to explain them during a conversation. In some cases this may be an attempt to show that they are medical "professionals," but it may also simply be a slip in communication. It is important for you to ask what terms mean without feeling embarrassed or ashamed, even if you ask two, three or four times. There is nothing shameful in wanting to know more about your child's condition, including learning new words that will possibly be used in the future. Some parents find it helpful to begin their own medical dictionary.

Communication of emotional, social or financial needs in a calm, matter-of-fact and non-judgmental way can help to assure that the medical staff is reminded of and will address more than just your child's physical needs. To promote optimal recovery at home as well as in the hospital, both you and your child should request assistance from members of the health team when you feel your needs are not being met.

FOR SIBLINGS

Open discussion of the illness with siblings is another area of concern for many parents. Siblings need to understand what is happening and why their family life has suddenly changed; the parents must decide how much information to share and whether or not to have siblings visit in the hospital. Talking about the illness provides opportunities for them to learn the facts, rather than fantasize or assume the wrong thing. When a child becomes ill, the entire family is affected, and the siblings need to still feel important. Chapter 7 details the benefits of open communication with siblings and describes how they can be affected by having a seriously ill brother or sister.

Each family communicates and expresses its love differently. When illness threatens the life of a child, one significant way you can offer support is by providing opportunities to discuss the illness with your child. This promotes a special parent–child relationship that offers benefits no other relationship can offer. Recuperative time spent in the hospital room or at home can be filled with loving and respectful conversations, rather than silence or mistrust. Time spent learning together, discovering new thoughts and feelings, creates a bond that can grow and be shared for a long time.

Parents sometimes blame themselves when their child becomes ill or is injured. The urge to blame someone or something is a part of the effort to rationalize what has happened. While parents may sometimes blame themselves for their child's illness, they may also forget or simply not realize, that they can perform an important role in the recovery process. A child diagnosed with a life-threatening illness is especially vulnerable to fear of the unknown and thus is more open to misconceptions about illness and hospitalization. Learning together and sharing feelings supports the child during this time of crisis.

In attempting to understand the diagnosis, it is important to remember that people have different ways of learning. This especially applies to children, who vary in their ability to express themselves and to comprehend new information. Often we must attempt to explain things through "trial and error" before a child may understand his illness. Depending on your child's age and developmental level, the illness may be discussed simply as being sick, or as a complex disease process. One thing to remember is that you are not expected to be an expert about the illness or child development. Your child's treatment team wants to work with and support you and your child through diagnosis, treatment and recovery. Physicians and medical personnel will provide information, but you are the most helpful in determining how much your child needs to and does understand. By openly communicating with your child's treatment team, you are better informed to help educate your child and understand his feelings.

The issue of communication will be discussed throughout the book. Depending on your child's age and level of understanding about the disease and hospitalization, different forms of communication may be necessary. The younger child can express many feelings through play (discussed in Chapter 4, therapeutic play). The older child and adolescent may need support from children the same age. Most important is that your child needs to feel informed, supported, and respected, but most of all accepted. Open communication by everyone involved promotes these feelings significant to a healthy recovery.

Notes

1. R. E. K. Stein, ed., *Caring for Children With Chronic Illness: Issues and Strategies* (New York: Springer Publishing Company, 1989).

2. P. R. Magrab "Psychological Development of Chronically Ill Children." In N. Hobbs and J. M. Perrin, eds., *Issues in the Care of Children With Chronic Illness* (San Francisco: Jossey-Bass, 1985), 709.

3. R. B. Darling, "Parent-Professional Interaction: The Roots of Misunderstanding," in M. Seligman, ed.; *The Family with a Handicapped Child: Understanding and Treatment* (New York: Grune and Stratton, 1983), 117.

4. L. W. Greenberg; L. S. Jewett; R. S. Gluck; et al., "Giving Information for a Life-Threatening Diagnosis," *American Journal of Diseases of Children* 138 (July 1984): 649–53.

5. G. Smith, "A Patient's View of Cystic Fibrosis," *Journal of Adolescent Health Care* 7 (1986): 134–138.

3

UNDERSTANDING YOUR CHILD'S REACTIONS AND BEHAVIOR

FEARS, FRUSTRATIONS AND
DEVELOPMENTAL NEEDS

THE CHILD AS AN INDIVIDUAL

We often admire the energy and imagination of the growing child. What makes each one so unique? Intellectually, children flourish by challenging their minds. Physically, they strengthen themselves through exercise, play and eating the right foods. Socially, they blossom by interacting with others. Emotionally, they develop by learning about trust, love, anger and compassion. A child develops in each of these areas by being with family and friends, playing alone and with others and attending school. Their experiences are like no others. Yet, when illness strikes, these avenues for learning are affected by the disease, its treatment, and the course of recovery.

A child's response to changes during illness may be based on "psychosocial" factors and personal resources available during the time of stress. Psychosocial factors can be thought of as attitudes, values, beliefs and emotional support that affect responses to the environment. Some responses are cognitive, a result of thinking through the experience and acting upon those thoughts. For example, a child finds his mother's favorite candy in the refrigerator and thinks "Well, I'll get punished if I eat Mom's candybar," and then puts it back. He then goes to his mother and proudly states that he was "going to," but *didn't*, eat it because he remembered it was her favorite. What happens? She hugs him and says "What a good boy, I guess you deserve a treat." He gets the candy bar anyway with a pat on the back. Other responses are emotional, based on the child's feelings. For instance, a little girl begins to cry in embarrassment when her sister laughs at a new outfit. Another type of response may be considered a "social" response, or behavior that is expected by others in society. Obeying rules in school is one example. The child who is ill may have one or all of these types of responses, depending on individual psychosocial factors and personal resources.

The treatment team often evaluates these resources in an attempt to understand the child's perceptions of and reactions to illness and hos-

PSYCHOSOCIAL FACTORS AND PERSONAL RESOURCES AFFECTING THE CHILD

The child's age and social experiences

The child's inner strengths, such as motivation, determination and developing values

Emotional support from family and friends

The parent's values and attitudes

The child's previous experience with illness or hospitalization

pitalization. The team may discuss them with you to understand your child a little better. You are a significant part of your child's life as you contribute to his development of values, attitudes and beliefs. Because of your knowledge of his experiences, you can help the medical staff anticipate and interpret your child's reactions to the diagnosis and medical care. For this reason, you and the medical team become "partners," and together you can provide the least stressful and most optimal treatment and recovery plans for your child.

When your child is introduced to a new environment such as a hospital, often he does not know how to behave. Previous attitudes and beliefs are challenged and often are difficult to apply to these new events. You may be there to offer guidance, but your child also relies on his own resources to cope with each new encounter and emotion. Although he has felt fear before, it may be very different this time. Pain caused by the illness and related procedures may be more intense than any felt before, and it may be perceived as threatening to his life and being. Separation from you and from friends may seem an eternity when the duration of the separation is uncertain.

One way you can help your child cope with these new feelings is to offer assurance that they will end. Your child's age and developmental level can determine the type of language you use. If you have a young child who does not understand minutes and hours, explain that a painful procedure will be over after a particular event, such as when the medicine is emptied from the syringe. If you need to leave for a while, you may say that you will return after dinner, for example. Setting a schedule often helps the child to feel more secure, but be sure to stick to it. No matter what the age, your child will often react more strongly if his fear of the unknown is not assuaged.

Medical staff are trained to understand possible reactions of children of various ages. Years of research and experience with hospitalized children have helped professionals to identify characteristic behaviors. Many believe that regardless of the illness, certain responses or behaviors can be expected, especially if the illness is chronic. Certain behaviors may also be expected based on a child's age and how he perceives the body. Children can view their bodies in several ways: through what they see or what they feel, through mental pictures of what they have previously seen, through symbols such as the valentine "heart," through previous learning experiences, or through fantasy.[1]

Children may cope with illness in any number of ways. Several common coping behaviors may include:[2]

- Asking questions
- Reducing tension by playing with other children
- Seeking comfort from others (wanting to be held) etc.
- Looking at or handling new objects
- Assuming responsibility for care
- Verbalizing feelings
- Attempting to gain control by preventing procedures or events
- Physical resistance or fighting
- Comforting self in solace or time alone
- Relieving tension through crying
- Acting out to get attention
- Seeking distractions (television, reading)
- Withdrawing from parents, avoiding others
- Regressive behavior
- Denying the illness
- Refusing responsibility
- Refusing to learn about the diagnosis or new procedures

Explanations of some of the behaviors you may see in your child are discussed below, along with suggestions for handling them. Once again, many factors affect why your child acts certain ways, but these are guidelines to help you understand some of them. Any concerns you have about your child's physical or emotional well-being should be discussed with your child's treatment team. Additional resources are discussed later in the book.

THE INFANT, TODDLER AND PRESCHOOLER

THE INFANT

The infant has developed little knowledge about illness, knowing only uncomfortable feelings of hunger, physical discomfort, and fatigue. When an infant is hospitalized, the new environment adds stress to the physical stresses already affecting him. Many variables of his life are temporarily, and perhaps permanently, changed.

In addition to separation from you, one of the most significant changes for your infant may be the general change in the environment. The infant four to eight months of age begins to acknowledge his surroundings.[3] The eyes focus on objects and people, absorbing images and differentiating colors and shapes. The sense of smell is very strong, and odors are noticed. In the hospital, the infant suddenly senses unfamiliar rooms, smells, people, and changed routines and becomes confused. You are the only stable thing in his life at this time, and he will react strongly when you are not present.

At times it may be necessary to leave your baby in the care of hospital personnel. Nurses are trained to understand the infant's feeling of loss and confusion and will comfort your child whenever possible. Toys or blankets from home sometimes help the child to feel more secure. Some parents feel better when a family member or friend the baby knows can stay while they go to work, do family chores, or simply take a break. Visits from siblings may also lessen the fear of abandonment. If children are not usually permitted to visit, your child's physician may be able to suspend the rules for a special visit.

Some mothers become that their babies may be more responsive or attached to nurses, in the same way a mother may be concerned about leaving a baby with a sitter while working outside of the home. It is important to remember that even physicians have commented that the mother "is the person who loves him, never pricks or hurts him and that she touches him in a different way which he recognizes."[4]

Even when you are present, your infant can be irritable at times. Attempts to comfort may seem useless, particularly during painful procedures. This is perfectly normal, as your infant is coping the best way he knows to—by crying. Because he may be concentrating on a specific thing, such as wanting to be at home with you or to be somewhere away from the pain, distraction may not always work. At other times, though, a distraction may seem to help as your infant searches for some outlet from the current stress, such as taking a walk or playing with a new toy.

Over time, you can learn how to help your baby by discovering his personal way of coping. If he just wants to cry, offer comfort. If you begin to feel upset, acknowledge your feelings. Everyone has a limit to the amount of crying he can withstand. It is normal to feel resentful to have such an unhappy baby, and some parents even find it difficult to "like" their infant. It is frustrating to spend so much time and effort comforting the baby and not be able to enjoy the smiles and triumphs of a healthy child. Although troublesome, and often resulting in feelings of guilt, these can be normal emotions from the stress of caring for a seriously ill infant.[5] Getting angry or frustrated, however, can increase tension and anxiety for the baby. Do not be ashamed about asking for assistance. The treatment team is there for support and they know you sometimes need a break.

Taking a walk with your baby may provide positive stimulation and a change of scenery. Perhaps you can offer a pacifier, favorite toy, or special blanket. If possible, rocking may prove soothing if nothing else seems to work. And as stated before, there may simply be times when he needs to cry to relieve tension and stress, or to cry himself to sleep. If your baby's cry changes (you know his different cries the best), and you become concerned, let the physician or nurse know. Changes you may notice include a constant, whiny type of cry; a higher pitched cry; or a more forceful cry. These changes may be simply the baby's way of saying that a new medication or food has made him uncomfortable, or they may indicate a change in the baby's health.

You may be able to reduce the stress of hospitalization if you inform the medical staff of your child's eating and sleeping routines.[6] Do not be surprised if your baby does not want to eat, however. Often the infant's appetite will be affected by the illness, the change in environment, and different treatments. Discussing his eating habits with the medical team may help them provide your baby with familiar foods, encouraging him to eat and get the nutrition needed during illness.

The use of pacifiers helps to meet sucking needs of young infants, even if they are not hungry. Infants receive gratification through sucking and exploring with their mouth, in addition to strengthening mouth and jaw muscles.[7] If the infant is not permitted to eat (such as before surgery), pacifiers become especially helpful when hunger stimulates the need to suck.

Following mealtime or bathtime rituals also allows consistency to promote trust in the environment, which in turn helps your baby to feel secure with other people. If possible, try to schedule these activities close to the same time as you would at home, and use a favorite bathtub toy, feeding spoon or bedtime pal or blanket packed for the hospital stay. Parents can also request that nursing care be done before the regular nap time if at all possible.

To continue developmental growth for your little one, take advantage of quiet moments to engage him in games of "peek-a-boo," "ten little piggies" or "I have your nose." Peek-a-boo helps an infant to understand how things disappear and reappear, thus helping him to cope with those times you must leave. Games like "ten-little-piggies" and "I have your nose" help the infant to learn about his body. Think of activities you do together at home and try to do them in the hospital room or playroom. By replicating some aspects of home life within the hospital environment, a basic sense of continuity may help your baby to more easily accept changes, although he will probably still have periods of crying and clinging.

A slow, gentle skin massage can also help your baby to relax, promote sleep and improve blood circulation. Begin in an area that is not associated with painful procedures (such as needle pricks). You can start at the toes and gently stroke or softly rub, making sure not to tickle. Work upwards toward the legs, to the back, and onward. You may find areas your baby prefers, and you can concentrate there. Eventually move toward areas that your baby may be protective of, showing him that they will not always be hurt. In addition to strengthening the emotional bond between you and your baby, massage helps him to develop an awareness of his body.

You may notice during hospitalization that your child reverts to behaviors characteristic of a younger age (termed regressive behavior). The older infant who no longer feeds by bottle may suddenly want a bottle again, or may want a pacifier not used in months. Regression to previous behaviors can be normal reactions as your infant searches for the security he has felt previously. As current stresses gradually decrease, and if his health status permits, the more advanced behavior will return.

The table below summarizes the typical fears and behavior reactions of the infant who is hospitalized.

Major Fears
Separation
Abandonment
Pain
Strange people
Strange objects
Loud noises

Behavior Reactions
Crying
Screaming
Searching for parents
Clinging to parents
Physical resistance (in older infants)

THE TODDLER

Many of the same stresses for infants also affect toddlers. Toddlers, however, are rapidly learning new, more advanced skills as they become more independent. Hospitalization is a major obstacle to learning the skills of walking, running, using hands and fingers and learning how to manipulate objects. The toddler is curious about how he can change the environment and how much control he actually has. This is demonstrated by your toddler's proud and determined statement of "No!" throughout the "terrible twos" and toilet training. Hospitals are a confining and restrictive environment that frustrates the toddler's need for freedom of movement. "The simple act of lying toddlers on their back can cause forceful resistance" and lack of cooperation.[8]

You can help during this time by offering opportunities for stimulating play. One example is stacking blocks. Your toddler will love building them up, then suddenly knocking them over. The object of play is not the finished project of a pretty tower, but the ability to demolish it. The child holds the "power" to decide if it stays or goes! Knocking down the tower also offers an acceptable outlet for frustration or anger.

The toddler also enjoys learning about new sounds and objects. A tape recorder, radio, musical instrument or pull toy offer chances to create change, either by making noise or moving an object all by himself. Additional suggestions are described under the section on therapeutic play, Chapter 4, which explains the importance of working out children's fears and frustrations with appropriate toys, including play medical equipment.

As your toddler learns about his physical abilities and the power to change things, he is also learning about good and bad. It is during this time that the concepts of "shame" and "doubt" are learned.[9] During toilet training the child learns that using a toilet is the right thing, while "messing" in pants is wrong. He may begin to feel ashamed when he understands how to use the toilet but still has "accidents." This becomes complicated during hospitalization, when medications and frequent administration of fluids affect bathroom habits. The older toddler requires additional support to understand that "accidents" are not his fault, and that he should not feel ashamed. He may be confused if his new ability and control are suddenly taken away.

Continue to explain that the medicine makes him go to the bathroom more and that it is okay if he has an accident. Some children are placed back into diapers to help monitor their urine and bowel movements. This can be very distressing to a child who is proud of just having learned to use the toilet. You should emphasize to your child that this is *not* punishment. Explain that once you return home, he can use the toilet again. It also may help to acknowledge other things he is doing well, such as applauding and giving hugs when he takes medicine or does something new. It will help to build confidence and lessen doubts about other abilities.

The toddler is also learning about controlling other behaviors. Temper tantrums and mood swings are normal but may occur more frequently during hospitalizations or even after returning home. This loss of control is very frustrating and your child may react with aggression and negativism. He does not want to be restrained or dependent upon you; he is torn between wanting his own way and wanting you to protect him. He may react by simply yelling "no," or he may even resort to physical aggression to regain control. Once again, supporting your child even during the "bad" times lets him know that you still love and support him. Tell him that you know how hard it is to sit still during a procedure, or that you understand that he does not feel well.

Some medications also cause mood swings. Prednisone, used to minimize inflammation associated with some types of surgery, illness and cancer therapy, is one medication known to cause such changes in mood. Some sedatives, anti-seizure medications or anti-nausea drugs may make some children more quiet or appear depressed. If parents learn that a medication may be affecting behavior, they may feel guilty about disciplining their child. Guidance and discipline actually help the toddler to feel more secure during this time of change when he is not sure how to act. Acknowledge feelings of discomfort, but be firm about what behaviors will be tolerated. It is difficult to set limits while your child is ill and has little control over the situation, but doing so reinforces the need for cooperation. A young child will adapt better to these changes if the parent does not alter his methods of discipline. Additional information on discipline is provided in Chapter 6.

Another aspect of development affected by hospitalization is the toddler's need for routine. He may be used to certain times or ways of sleeping, bathing, and use of the bathroom. Depending on your child's stage in development, disruption of routines may prompt him to revert to baby talk, needing a diaper, clinging or wanting the bottle. These are normal reactions to the stresses your child is currently encountering, and they should subside as the stresses decrease.

Toddlers do not yet understand how body processes work or how the body stays together. They often fear that their inside might come out or something terrible will happen to their insides when they are cut or pricked by a needle. This confusion may be caused by their interest in learning how to control their bowel and kidneys and in how some body fluids leave the body.

When toddlers are cut, they immediately seek to cover the wound, usually with a bandage. When a procedure such as a needle prick threatens to wound their skin, they will fiercely protest. This is a normal fear, not only of pain, but also of their body boundaries. Bandages help them to feel more secure about their bodies once they have been injured. Because they are unable to verbally express these fears, therapeutic play can help them to understand procedures and the healing process a little better, discussed in Chapter 4.

Your reaction to procedures also significantly affects your child's interpretation of the event. If you are calm and supportive, he is less tense and anxious. A big hug and kiss after the procedure also reinforces that everything is okay. If your child is feeling well enough, distraction after a procedure may help to minimize worrying about the new "boo-boo." Ask your child if he wants to hear a story or play a game.

Most pediatric units have special treatment rooms for procedures, separate from the regular hospital rooms, so that a child knows the hospital room where he sleeps is a "safe place." You can request that no procedures be done in your child's room if a treatment room is available. As a parent, and advocate for your child's well-being, do not be afraid to speak up. Your toddler will then maintain some sense of security, perhaps resting better when in his room. This also gives your child the secure feeling that there is a place in the hospital where he will not be hurt. The playroom is another room that should never be used for medical procedures.[10]

The list below summarizes some of the fears and behavior reactions of the toddler who is hospitalized.

Major Fears
Loss of control
Restrictions
Confinement
Dependency
Bodily injury
Shame
Doubt
Separation
Loss of routines
Strange people
Being alone
Loud noises
The dark

Behavior Reactions
Temper tantrums
Physical resistance
Aggression
Negativism
Regression:
    Soiling clothes
    Acting out
    Thumb sucking
Bad dreams

Depending on the extent of disease and treatment, and your child's personality, hospitalization can affect your toddler in various ways. By understanding some of his normal fears and developmental needs, you are able to facilitate coping, and in turn, a healthier recovery, by offering support, guidance, and learning opportunities appropriate to his age.

THE PRESCHOOLER

Like the toddler, the maturing child aged three to five is close to his parents yet at the same time he can be very active and eager to interact with the world. Confinement and fear of separation continue to be major stresses for this age group. Researchers have shown that young children do experience considerable stress in hospitals, yet they are more likely than older children to be reassured by parents and medical staff.[11] Because you are a strong influence, your reactions and attitudes can help determine your child's stress level as well as his level of cooperation.

A preschooler's demeanor, however, often belies his dependence on you; he might appear "quite mature and self-sufficient in usual activities of daily living and . . . begin to assume increasing responsibility."[12] Your "little adult" tries to cooperate all the while striving for acknowledgement of his growing independence. Sometimes, allowing him to make appropriate choices helps the preschooler to feel more self-sufficient. Perhaps ask your child what clothes he wants to wear (or, if a hospital gown is required, which socks, shoes or bedroom slippers he wants to wear). When hospital menus are distributed, ask your child to help choose meals for the next day. During bathtime, encourage him to wash as much as possible. Even if your child is receiving intravenous fluids in one hand, you can show him how to bathe with the other hand. This allows for some extent of control. If possible, let your child join in planning activities for the day, such as when to go the playroom (perhaps after bathing), or when you can play certain games. It helps to remind your child, however, that activities may need to be rescheduled if a procedure or treatment becomes necessary. By using a little imagination, you may find various opportunities for your child to do things that will boost self-confidence and maintain some feeling of control in this confining environment. In turn, you may be surprised at his willingness to cooperate.

Though we may often forget that these "little adults" are only three to five years old, we are reminded of their true stage of development during those wonderful and entertaining periods of fantasy and make-believe play. The development of a vivid imagination, in addition to the normal fears common to even healthy preschoolers, contributes to additional anxiety and misconceptions about the causes of illness, reasons for hospitalization and how various procedures or treatments are done.[13]

To help your child adjust to these new experiences in the hospital, it may help to show him the room, where everything is, and what equipment is there. If possible, explanations of what the equipment is used for can minimize scary fantasies. This may help diminish fears about the new environment. The next step is to introduce your child to nurses, doctors and other health professionals by name, so that they are more than mere faces. This can be a challenge even for parents, particularly in teaching hospitals where many medical personnel visit the floors. Do not hesitate to ask for names several times, and write them down for future reference.

Another way to help diminish fears of the unknown is to help prepare your child for treatments or procedures. Usually the treatments are explained in advance by a nurse or physician. Occasionally there may be a misunderstanding among staff as to who should explain a new treatment or medication to the family. If this has been overlooked, request that it be done. Once you have become familiar with the facts, you are then better able to help your child with questions he may be afraid to ask strangers. You are also more apt to pick up on certain feelings or behaviors that are not openly expressed. After the procedure, it sometimes helps to discuss feelings, but without dwelling on the negative aspects of the event (unless your child has a strong need to discuss them).

Most preschoolers are quite verbal, yet they may have difficulty expressing exactly what they are thinking. Play is a significant learning experience that also communicates many of the complicated and rapidly flowing thoughts they have. This is especially true for preschoolers who are unable to speak. These young children who are hospitalized, particularly with a confusing and frightening illness, benefit a great deal from continued opportunities to play and express themselves.

The preschooler may perceive illness in many different ways, but usually attributes its cause to something concrete, such as "bad cells" or germs "caught" from someone else. Children of this age group may also believe the illness is a result of something they did. Preschoolers are aware that events have causes but cannot understand the sequential steps or varied reasons leading up to an event. Their conclusions "are often based on what the child wants to believe rather than what he is told."[14] Discussing the "hows" and "whys" can alleviate some confusion but at times can even lead to other misunderstandings.

For example, one four-year-old began complaining of stomach aches. While discussing the importance of eating the right foods, she proudly stated, "You know why I'm *not* going to the bathroom when I have to . . . so I can keep food in my tummy and get big and strong!"[15] Here is an example of the need to discuss bodily functions, and the importance of nutrition with proper bathroom habits. After learning about why her body needs to get rid of "used" food, she returned to her regular bowel habits and the stomach aches stopped. This demonstrates how explanations may need to be repeated or discussed again in a different context.

Preschoolers frequently believe that hospitalization or painful procedures are punishment for "bad things" they did or imagined doing.[16] For this reason, it is best not to coerce your child into cooperating with threats such as "If you don't take your medicine the doctor will give you a shot." It is more helpful and less threatening to explain why and how certain procedures will be done. These explanations, even if they are not completely understood, will keep fantasizing to a minimum.

This is not to say that fantasy should be completely discouraged. Stimulating the imagination can actually help during and after procedures and treatments, if used appropriately. Coloring books about hospitalization or illness, as well as supervised play with medical equipment, encourage the child to express his beliefs and fears. Additional information is provided in Chapter 4.

Some preschoolers realize that being a patient has benefits such as increased attention and getting presents, and they may imagine new "ailments" to manipulate the situation. This behavior should be discussed and evaluated with medical personnel. It occurs particularly when parents decrease discipline and the child associates being sick with getting away with bad behavior. This type of "innocent" manipulation can develop into a trend that erodes the child's cooperation and increases his acting-out behavior. As explained in Chapter 6 (in the section of discipline), a parent's method of discipline should not change, unless additional guidance of the child's behavior becomes necessary.

On the other hand, some children try to convince parents that they feel better in order to avoid treatment. This tactic may come from fear or denial of the illness, or the child may truly believe that "magical powers" have made him well. Continued discussions about the illness and treatments will help your child to cope, and supportive guidance will encourage cooperation. Explaining the benefits of cooperation (i.e., "the sooner we can get through the procedure, the sooner we can go to the playroom" or promising a special treat, may also promote cooperative behavior. Over time, procedures and treatments for some children become easier as threats of the unknown diminish. Other children need help to get through the procedure, no matter how many times they have gone through it. Distraction tactics that are developed over time sometimes help, such as watching a toy or calmly humming a tune. Other suggestions are provided in Chapter 4.

The following table lists several ways you can help your preschooler during hospitalization and at the same time promote his developmental growth. By working with your child, you not only help him through a period of crisis but also prepare him for a healthy transition into school-age tasks and challenges. Your child may then feel better about himself and be more confident about his capabilities.

SUGGESTIONS FOR HELPING THE PRESCHOOLER

Let your child know that you are listening:
    Stop what you are doing
    Use eye contact
    Give answers specific to his questions
Offer opportunities for him to:
    discuss the illness, medicines or treatments
    express thoughts and fears
    exercise control, be independent—i.e. wash his face
    accomplish something new
    fantasize and play
Reward good behavior to encourage cooperation
Support angry outbursts with love and guidance
Praise efforts
Plan games or activities to do together

A healthy preschooler is assuming responsibilities for daily care (dressing, washing his face, feeding himself) and, in general, continuing to explore the world through play, questions and a very active imagination. All of these aspects of developmental growth are challenged by hospitalization and illness. You and the hospital staff can work together to promote continued progress in each of these areas. When your preschooler is given the chance to do things for himself, the positive feelings of accomplishment can help combat the negative feelings of dependence and doubt. Opportunities to play and interact with other children (when possible) also increase self-confidence and lessen the feeling of isolation.

THE SCHOOL-AGE CHILD

When a child enters school, once again a brand new world unfolds and offers him greater independence. Friends become new sources of support, information and emotional development as moral attitudes and values are established. Children aged five to seven may still believe, however, that they became ill or were injured as a result of bad behavior, and they may expect to get instantly better by taking one dose of medication or staying in bed for a while.[17]

Children aged six to 10 begin to better understand the relationships between events. Reality begins to replace the imagination as new knowledge is gained through a developing intellect and new social experiences. Your child realizes there are consequences for his actions and may be more conscious of his behavior. Learning to read and write expands intellectual curiosity as well.

When a child develops a serious illness at this age, he risks losing social contact with school friends and teachers, falling behind in schoolwork, and losing newly found independence from parents. You can help your child maintain contact with friends through phone calls, letters or even tape recordings. Arrange for him to do make-up work or new lessons while in the hospital if he is physically and mentally able. Fear of inferiority and failure also become prominent, and helping him keep up with schoolwork can reduce anxiety about falling behind. You might review math and reading skills with your child if he is interested. You can discuss schoolwork with your child's physician or nurse to ensure that homework would not be too stressful. Children requiring special education as a result of brain injury or a chronically debilitating illness will require special support. Additional information regarding school can be found in Chapter 4.

At this age, hospitalization and illness can be explained in more detail because the relationship between the two can be better understood. Fear of bodily mutilation remains strong at this age, but no longer as a result of fantasy, but a true understanding of pain and how procedures affect the body.

Your child is beginning to learn about body parts in terms of "usage and sensation."[18] Confusion occurs when he realizes that pain is part of the process of getting well, particularly if he had not been experiencing discomfort prior to diagnosis. To promote the child's continued sense of independence, it is important for him to participate in the scheduling of daily care activities. Your child will take great pride in helping to set his own schedule whenever possible. Children in this age group can become rebellious in an attempt to gain more control. Providing choices and allowing some control can help to prevent some negative behaviors.

The four- to seven-year-old begins to focus on one idea at a time, while a seven- to 11-year-old begins to classify things and compare them.[19] Competitiveness begins to show, and is one aspect of peer relationships that helps your child to develop satisfaction and accomplishment in interacting with others while evaluating his own actions. Because the school-aged child is more aware of others, your child may feel guilty about you or your partner having to leave home or miss work because of his illness. Offering support and acknowledging that no one is to blame helps to decrease this potential stress. The school-aged child with a life-threatening illness will also have the opportunity to socialize with other ill or disabled children. This can positively affect development by promoting feelings of empathy and respect for others. It has also been suggested that associating with others who are successful in dealing with similar problems can effectively support the development of a positive self-image."[20] "Normal" activities and interaction with healthy children, combined with hospital socializing, enables the child's continued development of self-respect, self-esteem, and a self-identity. While some parents fear the experience will have negative psychological effects, others feel that illness can actually help create a stronger and more empathetic person.

Several behaviors you may observe in your school-aged child as a result of these changes may include sudden temper tantrums, bed wetting, whining or clinging, withdrawing from you or others or refusing to go to school when he is able. The disruption of normal routines and increased challenges can be frustrating and frightening. Allowing time to absorb these changes and build tolerance to the experiences will help to determine which coping methods work best for your child. The negative behavior will then probably diminish as your child adapts.

THE ADOLESCENT

Young adolescents are becoming increasingly analytical and may understand that an illness may have several different causes and symptoms. If you have had the chance to learn about the disease or injury and how it is affecting the body, offer explanations and the opportunity for open discussions. These discussions can vary in detail, depending on your teenager's maturity, experience with illness, level of interest, and previous knowledge. Family conferences with the physician or nurse offer structured learning sessions where you can ask questions together. The mature adolescent should be treated as a young adult and allowed private discussions with the physician. Respecting this need for privacy can be important for the teenager's growing sense of responsibility for his own health. It also allows your adolescent to ask questions that are important but may be too embarrassing to ask in front of you or other adults. This can be important for the recovery process as he understands more about the body, or what activities he has been involved in or intends to participate in. These discussions also provide important information for the physician. The adolescent will also appreciate privacy for washing or using a urinal or bedpan. In addition it is very important that parents refrain from talking about their teen with other parents or patients in the hospital.

To feel more in control, your adolescent may want to know everything about his illness, including the bad side of it as well as a detailed account of the prognosis. Teens are particularly sensitive to what they perceive as dishonesty and distrust on the part of their parents, so open communication is especially important to maintain a good relationship. Communication between parents and adolescents varies from family to family. Some adolescents are more open about asking questions and talking about their feelings with parents, while others have a stronger need to keep thoughts and ideas to themselves. Parents also differ in how they discuss personal feelings, private thoughts or expectations. For this reason, no particular reaction or behavior can be termed "right or wrong," but each may be assessed as to whether or not it is helpful in the recovery process.

Some parents are very open and find it difficult when the adolescent appears to shut them out. Other adolescents may want to talk about sensitive subjects or even death, which may be uncomfortable for the parent. When needs seem to conflict with one another, it may help to compromise or seek help from support groups. For the adolescent who needs to talk, it helps to let him know that you will listen, and not be judgmental. Talking in a nonauthoritarian way also promotes open discussion. For example, saying "If you feel like talking, I'm here" may have more results than saying "You should talk about your feelings more, it's healthy for you."

Sit together when it is quiet, make eye contact, and simply show interest and concern. If you become uncomfortable, simply say you would like to talk further about your child's concerns but after you have had time to think about it. After you have been able to review your own feelings, or become better prepared by speaking with the doctor, nurse, social worker or clergy member, let your child know you are ready to talk again. If your teenager has been away from his friends for a while, the separation may give you an opportunity to become a friend rather than an authoritative figure. One study has shown that parents and health care providers were more important than friends in providing support for some needs of the adolescent.[21] If your adolescent loves to talk, simply begin by listening.

It may be, however, that your teenager resents being away from friends and as a result will shut you out or lash out at you. As hard as it may seem, try not to take it personally, and understand that he misses his friends and may feel out of control. Allow him time to prepare for visits, and give him time alone during visits and phone calls if it is appropriate. Respecting this need for peer comfort and support lets him know you recognize his independence. Tell him where you will be and when you will return, to assure him that you are still there for support. It may also help you to take a break for yourself.

Teenagers are eager to learn more about themselves and the world outside of the family. The need to learn about the illness and how it will affect their activities will vary from teen to teen.

Developmentally, the adolescent is establishing his own values, beliefs and attitudes. He is just beginning to try out various roles and to test adult coping strategies. While his personality begins to define itself, your adolescent is probably very sensitive to how friends feel about him. These factors, in addition to his current activities, groups of friends, and feelings about school and home life can influence how your adolescent reacts to hospitalization and illness. Some adolescents may show several of the following behaviors, while others may react very differently. The following are guidelines for understanding why some behaviors occur and why they can be expected during illness and hospitalization of the adolescent. They may occasionally be seen in younger children as well.

THE ADOLESCENT AND DENIAL   Denial is one coping strategy some adolescents use because they have thought of their previously healthy bodies as indestructible.[22] Some denial may be helpful in encouraging hope for recovery, but it must not interfere with treatments. The teenager's schedule should be reviewed with the doctor to determine what activities are safe during treatment. It is often difficult for the parent not to be overprotective even of children who are told they can be active. It may help you to realize that living as normally as possible helps to maintain appropriate developmental growth and continued peer support. A parent's overprotection often results in a battle of wills and can discourage the child from accepting needed support and understanding. On the other hand, your adolescent may need special guidance if he overcompensates with attempts to be "normal" like friends. If open discussions do not seem to help, encourage a private conference with the physician.

Sometimes your adolescent may appear to alternate between periods of denial and talking freely about the illness. This allows him some control over the situation, prevents overloading of information and helps to provide relief from being sick. Listen to specific questions when he or she wishes to discuss the illness, or join in a conversation about the fun things you did together on last year's vacation. If he appears to avoid discussing the illness all together, a little encouragement may bring to light any questions he may have.

THE ADOLESCENT FIGHTING FOR INDEPENDENCE Additional responsibilities, maturing values, and an expanding social life has your adolescent preparing for the big step of life on his own. When the adolescent is diagnosed with a life-threatening illness, he is torn between acting like an independent adult and seeking security and safety within the family.[23] Being a hospital patient increases dependence on others and often causes feelings of insecurity about one's physical self (his body is no longer "indestructable").

Angry outbursts can be a normal response to the stress of confinement and limited control. These outbursts are often directed toward the parent, who is perceived to be helping to enforce the necessary constraints. It can be helpful to support and accept this anger, while helping your adolescent to divert negative feelings to an appropriate activity.

Secretiveness and moodiness are other behaviors your adolescent may demonstrate in an attempt to gain control over his life. Moodiness can be related to hormone changes and medications, but it may be more evident when he feels out of control. Secretiveness may be expressed by periods of silence, private talks with friends, and engaging in activities without parental knowledge. These activities may be as simple as reading medical information, the Bible, or poetry or keeping a diary. In some cases, however, teens will engage in risk-taking behaviors. Some may begin to do things that actually are detrimental to their well-being or recovery, including experimenting with drugs and alcohol, refusing treatment or participating in dangerous activities.[24] This behavior may be an attempt to take control or may even be a sign of giving up hope for recovery. The teenager may feel that he wants to experience "everything" before dying. Participation in certain activities may also be an effort to maintain close bonds with friends.

Parents should continue to encourage discussions about what the adolescent is feeling or suggest participation in group activities with other teenagers with a life-threatening illness. Open discussions about the prognosis are important to define his expectations. If you suspect risk-taking behavior, it is important not to accuse without sufficient evidence. Dr. David M. Siegel, a pediatrician at the University of Rochester School of Medicine and Dentistry states that, "health care providers and family members must both educate chronically ill teens as to risks of experimentation, as well as anticipate and be somewhat tolerant of less than ideal behaviors."[25] This applies not only to chronically ill teens but also to those who have a life-threatening illness. Some parents often find it difficult to draw the line at certain behavior and to exercise discipline. If you feel the behavior is dangerous, it can be essential to your child's health to take action. Begin a quiet, private conversation by explaining that you respect his privacy. Ask if there is anything you can do to make things easier. Then in a matter-of-fact tone state your concerns about the need to listen to the doctor so there will be every chance for recovery.

If you suspect your teenager of negative behavior, simply but tactfully state why you think it is happening and offer a chance to explain. If an open discussion does not seem to help, then discuss your concerns with the physician. He may have additional suggestions or provide information on support groups that you or your teen may get involved in. Another solution is to draw up a "contract" between you and your child, thus allowing him greater control and responsibility. Contracts are discussed in Chapter 6. In general, discipline should be an expected consequence of negative behavior, but positive behavior should always be emphasized.

Offering opportunities to do things that your teenager has been wanting to do (that are safe and enjoyable) can help guide him onto the right track. It offers the opportunity for your teen to see how much he or she can actually do. Writing stories, poems, or music or learning new crafts are great outlets for expressing emotions and encourage a sense of accomplishment. Playing board games, pinball or video games are safe, "escapist entertainment. These outlets can be important for maintaining self-esteem and keeping up with peers.

THE ADOLESCENT WHO FEELS "DIFFERENT"   Missing school and social events and being away from friends create stress for your adolescent, who is becoming less dependent on you. Opportunities to maintain contact with old friends, make new friends at the hospital and participate in doctor-approved activities can be a big boost to morale. These can also be sources of stress.

Changes in appearance as a result of injury, medical treatments or procedures will make a teenager sensitive to being "different." Fear of friends' reactions may prevent your teen from attending social activities or maintaining contact with them, and this fear should be discussed. New clothing, a new hairstyle, hats and makeup, can help the adolescent to find new ways to present himself.

It is important not to force the issue of "fixing himself up" until your teen is ready, or he may be more apt to withdraw or feel self-conscious. If he indicates that he feels ugly or wonders how he will "ever be able to go out in public again," begin slowly by asking if he can think of any way to change his appearance. You can suggest that he talk with another adolescent in the hospital who has tried new things. Once again, peer support groups can be beneficial in these times of doubt. However, as two authors have stated, "Fears of being mutilated, disabled, and disfigured are all very prominent, and the honesty and reassurance that parents can offer can be the greatest help of all."[26]

Your adolescent may sometimes feel different when friends begin talking about their future or what they are planning to do over the summer. He may doubt his ability to establish a career, get married and have children, or maintain normal relationships. He may be concerned about lost opportunities to travel or establish a life away from home.[27]

Depending on your adolescent's specific diagnosis, prognosis and future treatment plans, several attitudes and behaviors may be seen. These include the "I don't care" attitude, resentment toward friends, avoiding school, or not following through on plans.[28] If your adolescent begins to distance himself from family and friends, appears depressed, refuses to go to school or declines to participate in favorite activities, it is very important to allow time for open communication. Your teen must, however, feel ready to talk about his feelings. Forcing a discussion may cause further withdrawal or create feelings of loss of control, frustration and anger. Once again, these issues should be discussed with your child's physician.

When your adolescent is ready to talk, tears may flow, an angry outburst may occur, or he may talk out everything calmly. Depending on feelings of stress, his interpretation of the situation and the future, and perceptions of available support, the adolescent can react in various ways. Simply offer support, encourage expression of these feelings, and, if necessary, discuss with the doctor the need for professional counseling. There should be no embarrassment in seeking counseling to help your adolescent through this difficult time. It is always better to have professional help before severe emotional stress hinders the potential for a successful recovery. An optimistic outlook lifts the spirits and can help even a bad situation seem more tolerable. Support groups are a great help in preventing feelings of isolation.

The adolescent experiences many changes in his body and in his life, and they are made more difficult to deal with by illness. Many of the typical difficulties parents have in communicating with adolescents are thrown a new twist. Fear of saying the wrong thing, and being too overprotective interfere with parental responsibility to guide the adolescent into adulthood. One thing to remember, however, is that now is a good time to establish and develop a stronger, closer relationship as the adolescent needs additional guidance. It is also important to remember the need for social support from friends outside of the family. A combination of family and peer support establishes a strong foundation for your teen to discover what he wants, needs and expects from the future.

SUMMARY OF BEHAVIORAL AND DEVELOPMENTAL ISSUES

Children of different ages react to situations in various ways. No one can determine how a particular child will behave or cope with stressful experiences, particularly during hospitalization for a life-threatening illness. Your child's age and developmental level will significantly affect how he perceives the world, how he learns, and how he expresses his feelings, thoughts and emotions. Based on years of experience and research of hospitalized children, health professionals have come to observe behaviors and coping styles commonly seen in particular age groups. These in turn are affected by the individual child's personality, life experience, and relationships with friends and family. As Baum and Baum have stated, "Although perceived by some to be more fragile than adults, children are often more flexible and adaptable than adults and often do far better in the face of misfortune."[29]

Notes

1. M. S. Steward, "Affective and Cognitive Impact of Illness on Children's Body Image," *Psychiatric Medicine* 5 (1987): 107–113.

2. S. Caty, J. A. Ritchie, and M. L. Ellerton, "Mothers' Perceptions of Coping Behaviors in Hospitalized Preschool Children," *Journal of Pediatric Nursing* 4 (December 1989): 403–10.

3. S. Maul-Mellot and J. Adams, *Childhood Cancer: A Nursing Overview* (Boston: Jones and Bartlett Publishers, 1987), 8.

4. C. Whittey and N. R. C. Robertson, "Parent–Infant Relationships in the Neonatal Intensive Care Unit," in D. Harvey, ed., *Parent–Infant Relationships,* Perinatal Practice Series, vol. 4 (New York: John Wiley & Sons, 1987).

5. D. M. Orenstein, *Cystic Fibrosis: A Guide for Patient and Family* (New York: Raven Press, 1989), 123.

6. Association for the Care of Children's Health. *Caring for Your Hospitalized Baby* (Washington, D.C., 1984).

7. Maul-Mellot and Adams, 8–9.

8. L. Whaley and D. Wong, *Nursing Care of Infants and Children* (St. Louis: C. V. Mosby, 1983), 866.

9. Maul-Mellot and Adams, 8–9.

10. Personal interview with Linda Ziegler, child life specialist, Johns Hopkins Hospital, Pediatric Oncology Unit, June 1989.

11. Personal interview with Dr. Brian Corden, pediatric oncologist, University of New Mexico School of Medicine, May 1989; Telephone interview with Dr. Donna Copeland, M.D., Anderson Cancer Center, Austin, Texas, May 1989.

12. Whaley and Wong, 867.

13. Whaley and Wong, 538.

14. D. B. Pruitt and M. Strickland, "Psychological Factors Affecting Children's Response to Medical Procedures: A Guide for Clinicians," *Psychiatric Medicine* 5 (1987): 199–208.

15. Personal communication, Jan. 14, 1990. Pediatric patient, Johns Hopkins Hospital, Baltimore, Maryland, January 14, 1990.

16. Maul-Mellot and Adams, 19.
Whaley and Wong, 868.

17. E. C. Perrin and P. S. Gerrity "There's a Demon in Your Belly: Children's Understanding of Illness," *Pediatrics* 67 (June 1981): 841–49.

18. Maul-Mellot and Adams, 9.

19. Maul-Mellot and Adams, 15–16.

20. M. M. Silverman and D. S. Koretz, "Preventing Mental Health Problems," in R. E. K. Stein, ed., *Caring for Children with Chronic Illness: Issues and Strategies* (New York: Springer Publishing Company, 1989).

21. M. A. Dragone, "Perspectives of Chronically Ill Adolescents and Parents on Health Care Needs," *Pediatric Nursing.* 16 (January/February 1990), 49.

22. D. W. Adams and E. J. Deveau, *Coping with Childhood Cancer: Where Do We Go from Here?* (Reston, VA: Reston Publishing Company, 1984).
National Institutes of Health, *Coping with Cancer: A Resource for the Health Professional*, Publication no. 82-2080 (1982), 76.

23. D. W. Adams and E. J. Deveau, 34.

24. Jane Brody, "Personal Health," *New York Times*, 2 November 1989, B20.

25. Jane Brody, "Personal Health," *New York Times*, 2 November 1989.

26. Adams and Deveau, 35.

27. N. Hobbs and J. M. Perrin, eds., *Issues in the Care of Children with Chronic Illness* (San Francisco: Jossey-Bass, 1985), 709.

28. Weitzman, "School and Peer Relations," 62.

29. B. J. Baum and E. S. Baum, "Psychosocial Challenges of Childhood Cancer," *Journal of Psychosocial Oncology* 7 (1989): 119–29.

4

HELPING YOUR CHILD

THERAPEUTIC PLAY

THE IMPORTANCE OF PLAY

When a child is hospitalized, one of his most significant means of learning is challenged: play. Children spend a majority of their time "playing," but in reality, play is a lot of work. It serves many important functions for the developing child,[1] helping him to:

- learn about his own body
- master new abilities
- socialize with other children
- become more independent
- learn to adapt to new situations, solve problems
- understand how things work (pushing, pulling, snapping together)

In addition to promoting growth and development, play in the hospital helps decrease regressive behaviors and can provide an outlet from the stress of treatments and procedures. At the same time, it gives the child the opportunity to learn about his medical condition and treatments and about the medical equipment involved. Playtime also provides an appropriate environment for working out frustrations and fears. It is very helpful for physically handicapped children, allowing them the chance to be more assertive or aggressive, and thus temporarily feel less dependent or helpless. Play is most therapeutic when it is initiated by the child and when he feels physically up to it. When adults lead games and activities, it may not feel like "play" for the child.

Some hospitals have professional child life specialists to help children to continue their developmental growth and cope with hospitalization through play. By asking questions and learning with your child, you can continue play therapy in the hospital room and at home. If your hospital has no such child life therapist, you can still provide the same opportunities and support.

THE CHILD LIFE SPECIALIST

Child life specialists are trained professionals that are available in some hospital play rooms to assist children during hospitalization. They also work with children in the privacy of hospital rooms if the child is confined to bed. They help to guide play activities that include "free or self-directed play" (where the child chooses play toys and initiates pretend play), medical play, games, crafts, and age-appropriate learning activities. They assist in preparing children for procedures and offer emotional support. They are also available to support parents in areas of development, communication and discipline. They can be a valuable resource for pertinent information on schooling, tutoring or special camps.

The child life specialist traditionally has a Bachelor of Science degree in psychology, child development or education and has completed an internship in a hospital environment (such as a playroom). The specialist is certified for his specialty and often trains assistants to work as a team. For hospitalized children, the child life specialist or assistant is a "safe" and "acceptable" professional that is non-threatening and often is perceived as a significant support person during hospitalization.

WORKING OUT FRUSTRATIONS

One aspect of play significant to the hospitalized child, or the child who is at home frustrated by illness or disability, is the opportunity to appropriately express fear, anger or loss of control. To help the child vent aggression and frustration, for example, child life specialists suggest that he play with Play-Doh, a punching bag, blocks, hammering toys or coloring books, throw objects into a bucket and that he be taken outdoors to play if a play area is available.

Child life specialists usually allow children to initiate play themselves and then help guide the expression of their feelings with the appropriate toys. If a child is willing, the parent or child life specialist may discuss feelings of anger or fear to help the child understand why he feels like "breaking something" or "hitting something." The child is also assured that it is okay to have these feelings. If the parent accepts these feelings and is comfortable about how they are expressed, they will understand and be able to control outbursts at home as well. Because of intense medical care and uncertainty of its outcome, the child with a life-threatening illness may be more prone to frustration and feelings of aggression. Providing an outlet through play activities in a safe environment helps promote healthier coping methods.

PLAY FOR THE INFANT AND TODDLER

When an infant is hospitalized, particularly for a life-threatening illness, sometimes the aspect of play is overlooked. The infant does not always show "active" forms of play, and parents may feel unsure of how to interact with their baby when he is ill or in pain. There are some activities that can help the infant during this critical period of development. A quiet time, after he is rested and fed and not in pain, is the best time to offer to play. Try not to overwhelm your infant with too much stimulation at one time. Based on your previous play experiences and trial and error efforts, you can offer one activity or toy at a time to see which one sparks interest. Allow your infant time to explore and play with each toy. Remember that he can become frustrated by seeing toys out of reach or hearing people without seeing them.

While infants are learning to control their little fingers and hands, small toys of different textures help them to learn about different surfaces. Stuffed animals, small rubber or plastic toys of different shapes, blocks and teething rings are excellent learning tools. Toys that make sounds, such as rattles and squeaky toys, help to develop hearing. Soft music can be soothing during fussy times or a happy tune can set the right mood for playtime. Babies are also fascinated by seeing their reflection in a mirror. If a baby-proof crib mirror is not available, take a walk to the bathroom and let your baby see both of you in the mirror. This can be a secure, refreshing way to play together.

To help stimulate the eyes, hang mobiles over the crib, place photographs on the sides of the crib, or display large drawings such as a bull's eye or face (with contrasting colors such as black, white and red). Very young infants, in particular, benefit from this type of imagery.

There are a few games that infants aged seven to 12 months particularly enjoy. One game that teaches how things can disappear and reappear is peek-a-boo. Peek-a-boo with surgical masks may also help your infant get used to seeing people wear them. Playing patty-cake also can help the baby to learn how to use his hands and make noise by clapping. "Ten little piggies" or "I have your nose" make learning about body parts a lot of fun. The nine-month-old and older infant also begins to express interest in putting items in containers and taking them back out again. Another fun activity—one that may be usually considered unsociable but has several benefits—is playing with food. This provides more opportunities to learn about textures, stimulates the sense of taste and encourages the child to eat.[2]

Bringing favorite toys or security objects from home also provides comfort and "reduces the feelings of strangeness and hostility about the hospital environment."[3] Using a little imagination and a lot of love, parents can offer many opportunities for play when the infant feels up to it. Helping your baby to develop his senses distract him from all the new, uncomfortable changes he is experiencing. To prevent infection or injury, frequently wash and examine his toys.

The young toddler can be difficult to entertain: his attention span is short and he has endless energy. You can engage his attention by rolling a ball, playing with dolls, using push/pull toys and playing with toys that open and close. Any activity that encourages the mastering of new skills such as walking, using his hands, or manipulating objects will usually be enjoyed. Just going for a walk for a change of scenery can sometimes help during fussy times. Physical activity, when possible, provides exercise that promotes sleep, improves circulation and often improves morale. If your child is unable to get out of bed, alternating toys and changing the scenery in the room and around the bed might prevent boredom.

The toddler may also benefit from therapeutic play with dolls that have a pretend intravenous needle, bandage, or similar medical device that he can relate to. Sometimes, teaching the child the name of hospital equipment and procedures will help him to become accustomed to some of the medical terminology. Even children as young as 10 months benefit from the opportunity to manipulate equipment, learning how it moves and what noises it may make.

PLAY FOR THE PRESCHOOLER

To provide the most appropriate methods for self-expression, learning and coping, therapeutic play is geared toward the child's age and developmental level. For the preschooler, the playroom is an excellent environment in which to learn about his medical condition. Considerations for parents include:

- allowing the child to assist with medical care and self-care (including toilet training)
- anticipating and accepting regressive behaviors (such as thumb sucking)
- allowing choices and control whenever possible
- encouraging exploration of medical equipment and new toys.

Some children are eager to learn about changing bandages, using feeding tubes, or learning how to work wheelchairs, walkers or other health care aids. Others need patient encouragement and support before attempting these tasks.

Communicating with your child to determine what he understands and wants to do can be achieved through therapeutic play. Playing with medical equipment, whether a model or real, helps the child to express his understanding of how procedures are done, how equipment works, and why it is necessary. Working through procedures step-by-step with dolls or models allows your child to express fantasy or "magical" thinking or to express any misconceptions about his illness (such as the concept of illness as punishment). For example, a preschooler may say to a doll: "And here is your IV, you have this because you were a bad girl."

It can also be very helpful for your child to continue with regular play activities, which promote a more natural atmosphere. These may include familiar activities from home and new games which provide choices *and* limits.[4] Playing with water, especially during bathtime, or playing with sand offer a welcome change. Emptying and filling containers helps your child to learn about how space is filled and can change. Creating a collage with stickers or building with blocks or Legos helps to satisfy the creative mind.

Suggestions for quiet play include listening to stories, allowing the child to tell his own stories, using puzzles for preschoolers, coloring, playing with dolls, dressing up, listening to music, playing with cars and trucks, practicing flash cards, listening to tape recorders, watching age-appropriate television shows, using Play-Doh, and cutting out pictures (if he is able to use preschool scissors). Providing opportunities for your child to have a sense of accomplishment and independence may help to boost morale and encourage cooperation. The child life specialist can assist parents in choosing appropriate toys and games for the child's particular medical condition and developmental level so that he will not become frustrated.

PLAY FOR THE SCHOOL-AGE CHILD

As your child matures, new issues arise from experiences outside of the home. The school-aged child with a life-threatening illness is confronted with new concerns about school and peers. To help the child during this stage of development, both developmental and hospital issues can be openly addressed during play. (See the following table.)

These issues can be addressed at various times, depending on your child's mood. Using role play, or acting out scenarios, sometimes helps the school-aged child to work out his feelings for a particular situation. Role playing is sometimes done during a group session in the hospital, where several patients can take part in different roles. If your child is willing, you can continue role playing at home. This may be particularly

ISSUES THAT CAN BE ADDRESSED THROUGH PLAY

Body Image: Interpretation of how he looks or how the body functions	1. Use dolls or medical equipment 2. Play dress up 3. Play games or make up games that label body parts, draw or color, read stories
Peer Relationships: Friends' reactions, changed relationships, new friendships	1. Go along with role play if initiated by your child 2. Provide opportunities for games, phone calls, visits, and play with others on the unit 3. Don't force your child to play with others
Separation: Fear of being left alone, new surroundings, death	1. Use dolls or medical equipment 2. Provide favorite toys from home 3. Peek-a-boo, games in which objects reappear (i.e. pop-up toys).
Dependence: Who to trust, fear of loss of control	1. Allow choices whenever possible 2. Allow anger or negative emotions in play 3. Let the child play the role of a doctor or nurse
Fantasy: Use in play, misconceptions about the illness or treatments	1. Use dolls or medical equipment 2. Let the child lead playing activities 3. Watch and listen to make-believe play 4. Draw, color, make collages, put on plays
Social Behavior: How to interact with others, being accepted	1. Go along with role play if initiated by your child 2. Play games with rules suitable for your child's age 3. Provide time, but don't force play with others
School: Returning, keeping up with the work, needing help, facing friends	1. Go along with role play if initiated by your child 2. Create games for learning math or reading skills 3. Read stories, talk about feelings regarding school

Impulsive Behavior: Coping with feelings, controlling emotions	1. Use dolls or medical equipment 2. Provide creative outlets: punching bag, water play, Play-Doh, throwing activities
Fear of the Unknown: The hospital, procedures, new faces, the future, pain	1. Go along with role play if initiated by your child 2. Use dolls or medical equipment 3. Look at hospital brochures or photo albums 4. Prepare your child for all hospital events

helpful when returning to school or when he has had a difficult time with clinic visits. Recreating the first day back at school and the reactions of other children can help to prepare your child for that big step in resuming a normal life. Role play is less stressful and less intimidating when it is initiated by your child.

Another way to initiate conversation may be to begin a card game, and casually ask about his day, ask about a close friend or comment on your child's good points. Sometimes watching a television show together may prompt discussions relating to his own life. Simply let your child guide the flow of the conversation, talking about what is important to him. Letting your child know that you are willing to listen will help to make it easier when he is ready to talk.

Remember, however, that the child still needs to have pure fun without being reminded of the illness all of the time. School-aged children like to compete, and a fun board game or guessing game can be a great morale booster. Research shows that social concerns have a high priority for school-age children and adolescents; they sometimes take precedence over fears about pain or hospital procedures.[5] Offering your child the opportunity to play with friends may be potentially stressful but can be reassuring as well.

WHEN THERE IS NO CHILD LIFE SPECIALIST

If your child's hospital unit has no child life specialist, seek assistance from child life specialists on other units. If there are no child life specialists at the hospital, you as a parent can perform their function by offering opportunities for therapeutic play and ongoing developmental growth as explained previously.

GUIDELINES FOR THERAPEUTIC PLAY

Allow your child to initiate play on his terms
Avoid criticizing aspects of play, as this will inhibit self-expression
Ask him to tell you about the activity or project
Provide real equipment (props are the next best thing) for medical play
Provide opportunities to work out frustrations and fears
Periodically change toys or activities to prevent boredom, allow personal choices
Select challenging toys that provide opportunities for achievement but are not frustrating
Encourage physical activity or play outdoors when possible

Even though you may not have had the training of a specialist, no one knows your child better than you do. You will have an idea of the more enjoyable and educational activities for your child. Following the suggestions for toys and activities, with guidance from your child's doctor, you can provide the same support for your child. You can ask the nurse or doctor for unused syringes (without the needles), Band-Aids or bandages, tongue depressors, etc., to help with medical play. Using one of your child's dolls, have your child pretend to be the doctor or nurse doing a particular procedure. This can help you understand how your child thinks intravenous needles work, why needles are needed, or whether or not he understands why they are necessary to get better.

If your child requires surgery and no one has offered a tour of the operating or recovery rooms, simply request one. If you are not permitted in the treatment room when your child requires procedures, ask if you may familiarize yourself with the room so you can be prepared for any questions your child has.

Even without the assistance of a child life specialist, your child can more easily accept his illness and hospitalization with guidance from the person he trusts the most: his parent.

OTHER WAYS TO HELP

There are numerous ways parents can be involved with their child during hospitalization. Play is a major form of communication for children and can help parents understand some of their child's feelings. One area that is more difficult to address is helping your child to cope with pain.

DEALING WITH PAIN

When a child is in pain, or is forced to endure a painful procedure, it is difficult to determine how he will first react. Your child's interpretation of the pain may be based on how sudden the pain is, why it is happening, how long it will continue, if it will return, and past experience with pain.[6] Once your child has demonstrated a particular behavior or coping style, you and the treatment team may come to expect similar patterns if the procedures must be repeated or if the child has continued bouts of pain. Some children always follow similar coping patterns, and some change them as they learn new ways to cope. Only time and experience will tell how your child will ultimately react.

Pain is an individual experience and each person has a different tolerance level of pain. One study has reported that 18 children undergoing the same five painful procedures for leukemia varied as to which one they felt was the most painful. Their conclusions also differed from what the health professionals expected would be the most painful. Parents can best understand their own child's experience during painful procedures and thus communicate their child's fears and perceptions to the health care workers. In turn, parents can help find coping strategies that work for their child.

The child can be prepared for painful procedures, treatments or surgery with discussion of possible "sensations" and ways those "sensations" will be alleviated (such as medication). While being honest promotes trust between you, your child and the medical staff, the words you choose to describe how or what your child may feel can affect his level of anxiety and his perceptions of the pain once it occurs. Suggestions for appropriate words are discussed in Chapter 2 (see "The Importance of Communication"). If the procedure is fairly brief (such as inserting an IV) and is done while your child is awake explain what will happen during the procedure and how long it will last. This can prepare your child emotionally to cope with the event.

To help children through procedures and treatments, some hospitals have found success with distraction games, fantasy or imagery. Depending on the child's willingness, some children imagine themselves floating on a cloud, being on the beach, riding a boat or being a brave hero immune to all feelings of pain and fear. This technique can teach the child to master pain rather than avoid it.

Sometimes children cope well by concentrating on counting during a procedure, quietly humming, or focusing on an object—a technique similar to that of the Lamaze method used during childbirth. At other times children have used headphones and listened to music to distract themselves. Another calming technique is to sooth your child by stroking his hand or back. If nothing else works you can try to have the child focus directly on the body part and what will be happening.[7] Some children simply do best by crying. Reassure your child that this is okay. Children vary in the way they cope. By working with your child, you can help find ways to tolerate painful experiences.

For chronic pain, some have suggested combining imagery with rhythmic breathing, concentrating on even, easy breaths. Progressive muscle relaxation may also help. Start at the toes, relaxing them, then the legs, the abdominal muscles, the arms, the hands, and then the neck. A child can take great pride in learning to control the amount of tension in his body through breathing.

Often parents have already discovered their child's own methods of coping from previous illnesses or painful experiences. If this is the case for you, remind your child about what has helped before and tell the treatment team about his personal way of handling pain. In one case, a three-year-old boy would only cooperate with an injection if he was allowed to scream until the needle was removed. Screaming was his way of relieving tension and distracting himself during the injection. The nurses simply put cotton in their ears and closed the treatment door tight. The little boy held still the whole time while screaming. After the needle was removed, he did not even whimper (as long as a Band-Aid was placed over the injection site). Simply support your child by accepting and encouraging his way of coping, as long as it does not interfere with a procedure or the administration of medication.

PREVENTING AND OVERCOMING FEAR
GENERAL FEARS

Fear can be a normal part of growing up. While anxiety is defined as an uneasiness or apprehension, fear is defined as "an unpleasant often strong emotion caused by expectation or awareness of danger".[8] Thus fear is a much stronger emotion in response to a real or perceived threat and actually creates changes in the body, such as a rapid heart beat, nervous energy, and sweating. These changes help prepare the body for confrontation of fear or for escape.

In addition to the obvious need to minimize a child's emotional distress, helping a child to overcome fear also protects his physical condition during illness, when the body is already compromised. Reducing fear also can foster cooperation with procedures, taking medication, or daily care.[9] Depending on the circumstances, however, some believe that "anxiety and fear are not in themselves bad. In fact, anxiety and stress can be strong motivators for further growth and development."[10] In fact, these emotions may prove beneficial in helping to foster cooperation.

As previously stated, even healthy children develop fears from an active imagination combined with the lack of experience in the world. Older children may have fears based on previous experiences or on things they have heard, read about or perhaps even witnessed. Responses to fear will vary, depending on the child's perception of how threatening the feared situation or object is, how suddenly it occurred, how the parent is reacting, whether or not there is a way to escape or stop it, whether or not the child has developed a way to cope and whether or not he can be assured that the fearful experience will actually end.

Increased anxiety or a sense of helplessness often are a result of feeling out of control and being unsure of what to expect. One way to help your child with these feelings is to set schedules whenever possible. Picture charts are a fun way to show when routines such as meals, baths, naps, medications, playroom time or special activities will occur. Have your child place stickers on the chart or mark a box on the chart when each event occurs. When an unpleasant procedure is required, perhaps plan a special treat afterwards to help him feel better about going through with the procedure.

Sometimes parents and medical staff can prevent or minimize potential fears. Unexpected and unpredictable events, noises, touch, pain, and even sudden movements can startle the unprepared child and initiate a fear response. The very young child and infant are more affected by these types of unexpected situations. Moving slowly and deliberately while speaking softly is more predictable and soothing. When a noise is expected, gradually move the origin of the noise toward your child or infant, or if possible soften the noise at first. If your child is old enough to understand, you and the medical staff can prepare him by explaining:

- Where he will be touched
- What he may feel (pressure, warmth, tingling, etc.)
- What he will hear
- What he will see (what the equipment is, and what it is used for)
- What will happen (steps of the procedure).

It is also helpful to give your child the opportunity to explore the hospital environment. Many hospitals now provide tours of operating rooms prior to scheduled surgery so your child knows what to expect and can ask questions.

Regardless of how much we try to prepare children, we can never alleviate all of their fears. The next best thing is to help them to overcome the fear and cope with the situation. Just as we provide information to help prevent fear, continuing to explain and reinforce positive outcomes will help your child to adjust when he does become fearful.

Teaching the child to control some aspect of the situation whenever possible builds his confidence and trust. School-aged children in particular learn to deal with fears and anxieties by acting them out.[11] Therapeutic play is one such outlet.

Allowing your child a degree of control also promotes coping. For example, whenever it is possible, let your child decide what position to be in (lying or sitting), let him make choices about his surroundings (such as whether to listen to music or have quiet time) or let him decide when the procedure will happen. This may be more feasible at home than in the hospital environment. A little creative imagination of your own, listening to your child's requests, and working with the medical staff may provide a better way for your child to overcome the fear.

One additional way to help diminish fear is to show examples of how others have successfully endured a situation, particularly if they were the same age as your child. For example, a child who is to receive an intravenous treatment may be less fearful if he has seen children who already have an IV playing on the unit. Talking to the other children may also help to reassure him.

FEAR ABOUT CHANGES IN THE BODY

Many fears and anxieties relate to changes in body appearance. Children of different ages have different feelings about their bodies. Their reaction to physical changes may be based on previous exposure to others (such as older people who have become wheelchair bound), images of handicapped people on television, or their own experience of the normal changes of adolescence. Children who are physically changed as a result of an illness, injury or treatment develop a new perception of what they consider to be normal for their own body.

Some children who have required medical care for some time may fear being separated from medical equipment that they have been connected to.[12] A child may begin to think of tubes or other devices that have been attached to his body *as* part of his body and may fear that because the equipment has been so closely linked with bodily functioning, his body will not work properly without it. Parents can help their child cope with this separation by explaining when and why the equipment or medical device will be removed.

As previously explained, younger children fear any injury to their body. This is due to their lack of understanding of how the body stays together and how it heals, as well as to their active imaginations. Younger children are comforted by quickly covering wounds with Band-Aids or bandages "to make sure the blood won't run out." They also need to talk about the new "boo boo," seeking reassurance that the body will not continue to change, or that they will not die from what has happened.

Distraction sometimes help the younger child, depending on the circumstances. Younger children may also overcome a change in their bodies more easily than older children because their body image is still being formed. For example, a young child who has undergone amputation of a limb may quickly adapt and compensate by learning how to use other parts more effectively.

School-aged children are also very concerned about being hurt or experiencing changes to their bodies, but on a more practical level. They are at a point in their lives when they are just beginning to socialize, finding out how they fit in with others and what they are able to do. Changes that may affect school-aged children the most are probably those that affect their ability to master new skills or do what other children can do. Helping your child to continue with creative and academic efforts, and emphasizing his strengths and abilities, can make it easier for him to accept changes.

Adolescents are very concerned about being accepted by friends and becoming independent of their parents. They can be emotional and very sensitive as a result of hormonal changes and the development of sexual characteristics. Some feel that adolescents are more fearful about bodily changes than the threat of death. Modesty and sexuality are prominent concerns, and these can be strongly affected by illness and hospitalization. As explained in Chapter 2, parents can provide support for their teenager by allowing him privacy. Health professionals may, at times, need to be reminded of these concerns. Your child may be very appreciative if you remind nurses and doctors that he needs a curtain or door closed, or even if you stand behind the curtain yourself. School-aged children and adolescents vary in their need for privacy and the need to have a parent present. Other major concerns of older children include providing information, being truthful, offering respect, and providing the opportunity to do self-care. Accommodating these needs when possible will provide the support your child needs.

FEAR ABOUT DEATH

Another area that parents usually have difficulty discussing with their child is the fear of death. Most parents wait for the child to bring up the subject, in an effort to protect him. As mentioned in Chapter 1, the possibility of death should be discussed openly and honestly with the child if he appears to be concerned about it. If a child asks if he is going to die, one way parents can find out more about his child's fear of death is by asking in return, "Do you think you're going to die?"[13] Children of different ages have different concepts of death, its finality and how it will happen. Parents can only understand if death is a concern if they provide opportunities for their child to discuss it. If a child on the unit has died, or if a television show depicts a child dying, observe your child's reactions, offer time for your child to ask questions and listen to comments he may offer that may indirectly relate to himself.

Infants and toddlers do not have the ability to understand death but strongly fear separation. Parents can reduce the fear of abandonment by being present whenever possible, providing security toys from home, placing snapshots from home on the bed or crib, or having someone the child knows visit when the parent cannot be there. Frequent touching or cuddling is also very comforting.

Preschool children also do not fully comprehend the finality of death and may believe medicine or special care can bring them or others back after dying.[14] They may associate sleep with death and may become fearful of having an operation or even falling asleep in the hospital. If they need medicine that makes them drowsy or sedates them, they may need reassurance that they will awaken after their body has rested for a while. Ongoing discussions about how and why procedures are done and how pain will be alleviated will all help to diminish fears about death by minimizing fantasy.

School-age children are better able to comprehend the finality of death yet may still have difficulty believing it can happen to them. They still may wonder about it, however, and become very conscious of any bodily changes that remind them of the possibility.[15] They may need to talk about it, sometimes out of curiosity and sometimes to seek reassurance about their understanding of what is happening to them.

Adolescents are deeply involved with establishing themselves as individuals and as part of a group of friends and with planning for a life of their own. They usually understand death at an adult level and can become very concerned about the risk of dying before they have experienced everything they wish to explore. Teens have the strong need for honesty and to have their feelings respected, and open discussions are essential if they begin to talk about the possibility of their own death. Parents, health care workers and clergy members can all help the adolescent work through these emotions, especially if friends feel awkward or scared about these discussions. When the possibility of death exists for a teenager, it makes him different from his friends and changes how he views future plans. Providing time to talk about death when your teen openly expresses the need can provide an important opportunity to work through feelings that affect how he copes with an illness or injury.

The hospital environment is a busy, noisy, strange new world for children. Helping them to prevent or overcome fear during hospitalization lessens tension and stress, thus allowing them to rest more and giving them a better chance to recover. After release from the hospital, the parent should continue to respond to these concerns in the home environment.

ONGOING TREATMENT

Parents may find new concerns when children require ongoing medical care after returning home. The following discusses some of these concerns and suggestions for helping your child after discharge from the hospital.

EFFECTS OF CONTINUED TREATMENT ON BEHAVIOR AND MORALE

Children who require intermittent hospitalizations or clinic visits for ongoing treatment are affected to various degrees. To understand how their child might feel, parents should consider the purpose of additional care. Will most visits be routine therapy or a result of complications of the illness or therapy? Will there be repeated painful procedures? What is the frequency of scheduled visits and expected duration of the treatments? Each of these can affect a child differently and must be considered.

Hobbs and Perrin suggest that as the illness becomes chronic, and perhaps when treatment must continue over time, the child may require additional support and guidance in eight emotional areas.[16] An example of these needs, as defined by Hughes, and how to deal with them are shown in the table below. According to Hughes, the needs will change with the child's developmental growth and the status of his health. As circumstances change, certain needs may take priority over others. By listening to and watching your child, you should become familiar with his way of communicating what emotional needs are important at any given time. It may be comforting to remember that these are needs shared by the healthy child as well.

Research in the 1970s and 1980s mostly focused on the negative consequences of severe and chronic illness.[17] Recent research, however, proposes that psychological problems of seriously ill children are less prevalent than originally stated.[18] Families that feel overwhelmed by the experience have been found to adapt and cope better by obtaining pro-

EMOTIONAL NEEDS OF THE ILL CHILD	*CONSIDERATIONS FOR PARENTS*
Love and affection	Your child needs to feel these are unchanged, provide whenever possible, avoid letting frustrations get in the way
Security	Your child may have increased anxiety about bodily functions, financial burdens on family, or loss of employment by a parent. Provide time to discuss these fears.
Acceptance	Your child may fear changes in his relationships. He may also become bashful around strangers. Provide time with friends, demonstrate trust in health professionals.
Self-respect	Your child may need support in the areas of self-esteem and self-confidence. Allow privacy, acknowledge achievements, minimize overprotection or overindulgence.
Achievement	Your child may become anxious about an extended absence from school. Encourage contact with peers and teachers.
Recognition	Your child may lack confidence in his abilities. Acknowledge new skills and accomplishments, focus less on the illness, and allow self-care when possible.
Independence	Your child may feel a need for increased independence. Provide time with friends, as well as opportunities for self-care when appropriate.
Authority and discipline	Your child may need special guidance during illness when he's not sure how to act. Do not change discipline techniques if possible, be firm when appropriate.

fessional help or joining support groups.[19] Research has also shown that children who recognize and accept restricted activity and physical limitations tend to adjust better.[20] When a child incorporates these changes into everyday routines, treats limitations as a new way of life and focuses on his strengths and abilities, he will be less apt to get angry or frustrated. Acceptance by others, satisfaction with recovery and eventual progress may depend on how much he interprets the changes as a "handicap." Discussing the reasons for any limitations helps the child understand and accept them. By providing the child with continued opportunities for developmental growth, and new achievements, you can also help him to find more satisfaction out of life.

CLINIC VISITS

As with most experiences, children and parents vary in their feelings about and responses to ongoing evaluation or treatment in a hospital or clinic. Some feel they are being constantly reminded of illness just when they are attempting to normalize their lives again. Others view it as a step toward final recovery yet are apprehensive about finding something wrong again.

Children with cancer often become anxious before clinic visits in anticipation of painful procedures or medications that make them feel ill. These children require support for the ongoing visits and benefit from learning appropriate coping strategies. Often older children find reasons for not going to the appointment or parents have difficulty in getting the child ready to go. Open and ongoing discussions about the purpose of the visit, what it entails, and how it may make the child feel are all important to maintain trust with the child. Pretending to go somewhere else will only create undue resentment and fear for the child upon arriving at the clinic. Reminding your child of the benefits of going to the clinic—explaining, for example, how treatment will help keep the disease in remission (and *then* no more clinic visits)—may help when he feels discouraged.

Children returning for the first follow-up exam (such as for burns, trauma or diabetes) need special reassurance. They may fear the same painful experiences they experienced in the hospital. If they question what will happen and you are unsure, call beforehand and request information from a nurse or the doctor. If both you and your child are prepared, there will be less tension and fear of the unknown.

For younger children, bringing along a favorite toy or activity often helps during the anxious moments you must often endure in the waiting room. It is important to tell your child about the visit beforehand, but usually only the day before or the day of the visit so that he will not become too anxious. If a clinic visit will interrupt other plans or scheduled activities, it is helpful to explain this to your child ahead of time.

Repeated procedures have their benefits and disadvantages. Fear of the unknown is somewhat removed, and thus there should be less anxiety about what will happen. If the procedure is painful, however, repetition of the pain may affect feelings of control and may make the child fear he is not getting well. Once again, it is important to discuss with your child how he is feeling and to observe how he reacts with each visit. Any concerns about the child's morale should be addressed to the physician so that he can make changes if possible.

If your child begins to seem depressed or withdrawn or actively protests visits, several activities may help:

- A calendar chart that counts down each scheduled visit. It is important to remind your child, however, that the number of visits is subject to change based on his health status.
- Doing a favorite activity or visiting a special place after each visit
- Planning a special vacation with the physician's approval
- Having siblings accompany your child

It is important to remember that there should be a balance between the child's needs for medical care and the need to continue with normal activities. Provide opportunities for creative activities of his choice. "Allowing at least some self-direction helps to keep up morale."[21]

In 1981, a program was developed by the National Kidney Foundation to prepare youngsters for adolescence and to offer suggestions and discussions regarding daily experiences of dating, social interactions and seeking new jobs (see Appendix A, National Kidney Foundation). Depending on your child's illness or injury, local organizations or foundations may help you initiate a similar program.

RETURNING TO SCHOOL

A major source of stress for many children when they come back home is the return to school or enrollment in a new "specialized" school. Several issues may need to be addressed in order to provide a comfortable transition for your child.

ADAPTING TO SCHOOL: PHYSICAL, EMOTIONAL AND MENTAL STRESSES

Remember your first day of school when your palms were sweaty and your heart was racing? To some extent, a child who has missed school, particularly for a life-threatening illness, may have similar feelings upon reentering school. If your child has missed more than one or two weeks of school, has any visible physical effects from medications or procedures, feels physically weak or will continue to miss school for clinic visits or additional hospitalizations, his school life has surely changed. Your child will probably worry about how the teachers will treat him, but above all he will worry about his friends' reactions.

"School phobia," or anxiety associated with school, can be a very normal reaction to the changes caused by a life-threatening illness.[22] If you try to understand your child's perceptions of the illness and how it has changed his life, you can better understand why he fears school and how he must adapt to the changes in school life. Many children look forward to returning to school, while some need encouragement and more support. Your child's personality, adaptability, perseverance, social skills and peer support all have an impact on how he will adjust.[23]

Various physical, emotional, and mental stresses may affect your child's adaptation to the school environment. The table on page 70 lists the stresses as well as the benefits of reentry.

Some children expect to feel "back to normal" upon returning home and to school. Discussions about how your child can expect to feel can help minimize the frustration and confusion he may feel when he experiences periods of fatigue or weakness.[24] Depending on your child's developmental level, he may be affected to varying degrees by his previous involvement in athletics, his particular illness, and any side effects from medication.

Some illnesses or treatments may permanently affect a child's memory, ability to concentrate or ability to learn advanced skills. In these cases, the parent can be a strong advocate for his child in working with health and education professionals to find the most appropriate yet challenging educational resources.

There are numerous federal programs that offer services to chronically ill children. These include Head Start; Early Screening, Diagnosis and Treatment; The Social Sciences Grant; Title 5 of the Social Security Act; and community health centers. A social worker or local community center may be able to provide you with specific information relevant to your child's needs, especially if treatment is ongoing.

TEACHER AND PEER RELATIONSHIPS

School-aged children and adolescents become increasingly concerned about their friends' approval and acceptance as they begin to value the emotional support of children their own age.[25] The desire to succeed, to keep up with peers, and to please teachers may create concern about

STRESSES AND BENEFITS AT SCHOOL

STRESSES AT SCHOOL

CAUSES OF PHYSICAL STRESS	CAUSES OF EMOTIONAL STRESS	CAUSES OF MENTAL STRESS
Fatigue, lack of energy	Self-centeredness	Difficulty concentrating
Handicaps	Decreased social	Academic achievement
Appearance	interaction	ment
Athletic abilities	Preferential treatment	Side-effects of medications
Sexual development	Others' expectations	cations
Side-effects of medications	Peer acceptance	Make-up work
cations	Personal motivation	
Increased risk of infection	Flexibility	
	Attitude toward school	

BENEFITS OF SCHOOL

PHYSICAL BENEFITS	EMOTIONAL BENEFITS	MENTAL BENEFITS
Exercise	Independence from home	Intellectual stimulation
Increased stamina	Peer interactions	Distraction from illness
	Reassurance of abilities	Educational opportunities
	Sense of purpose	nities
	Increased confidence	
	Development of self-concept	
	Development of social skills	
	Less isolation	

how the recovering child may be treated when returning to school. This need to socialize and be part of a group outside of the family is part of the normal process of developing self-esteem and an identity in the community.

Concerns about returning to school may be influenced by several factors. Your child's attitude toward school, changes in his appearance, involvement in school activities, relationships with friends and teachers, and your attitudes and concerns all have an impact on his state of mind. This is particularly true when the illness has been sudden.

One way the parent may help is to contact one or several teachers from school. Some teachers appreciate information about the child's medical condition. It helps them to have realistic expectations about the child's health, attendance and performance in the classroom. Perhaps begin by arranging a meeting among the teachers, health care team and the family, or by phoning teachers or counselors who will be working with the child when he returns to school.[26] Discuss what should be expected of your child, and stress that the teacher should continue to treat him as normally as possible. Offer to explain the medical condition and its treatments so that the teachers may share this information with the students, who in turn may react more positively when they know more about the illness. Periodic meetings or phone calls after your child has been in school for a while will keep everyone up to date on his condition and changing needs. You also need to be informed of your child's exposure to any communicable diseases (such as chicken pox) if his immune system has been weakened by medications or the illness itself.

If a local organization has pamphlets or visual aids about your child's illness or disability, teachers may wish to distribute them to the class and review the information during a "question and answer" time. This reinforces factual information and cuts down on conjecture about the disease process or treatments. Teachers should be careful, however, not to "label" your child, as this may "handicap" him with certain expectations and can make him feel different from his friends.[27]

Some recovering children use their new-found knowledge about an illness or medical procedures to write essays, present class discussions or to "show off" a new vocabulary. Explaining the illness, particularly the painful aspects such as a change in appearance or going through treatments, sometimes instills empathy among peers and discourages teasing.[28]

Teasing is of course one aspect children fear they will encounter upon returning to school. Preparing your child for this type of reaction may help him develop ways to cope. Parents sometimes suggest that the child initiate jokes about himself, not with self-deprecation, with a positive attitude. In this way, the child shows that he feels comfortable with himself, and this positive self-image will influence the attitude of his peers.

Children who do tease may do so for various reasons. These may include ignorance about the illness, fear of catching the illness, confusing the illness with another disease, or attempting to show some control over the ill child. Explain to your child that his reactions to the teasing can help to promote or lessen it. If he is calm and does not react, he takes the fun out of being mean. If he cries, fights or yells back, his response may bring on even more teasing.

It helps to talk with your child about how he feels about school, what is happening at school and how others are reacting. If your child is having a difficult time reentering school it may help to join a support group or speak with a therapist. School should be a place for learning, socializing with friends and working toward the future. It should not be a tormenting, fearful experience. As your child's advocate, speak to teachers, the principal and other parents if necessary. Older children should be consulted before you intervene, however, as they often try to resolve their own problems and may feel embarrassed or out of control if you try to help them.

ABSENCE AND ACADEMICS

As shown in the table on page 70, there are several sources of stress for the child returning to school. Mental stress is sometimes easy for a parent to overlook until it is reflected in a child's schoolwork and report cards. Absence from school is a main contributor to lower grades and must be monitored to determine special needs for tutoring, repeating a grade, or attending a special school. The physician, nurse or child life specialist may help you to understand what should be expected regarding school, based on your child's illness, health status, recovery process and need for continued treatment. If your child's illness affects attendance, it is worthwhile to discuss with the doctor, social worker or child life specialist the need for tutoring or tele-teaching services, which may be available from public services in special education. Tele-teaching incorporates the use of a television and phone in the child's home that is directly linked to the classroom so he can observe the teacher and class, and can participate using the phone. Counseling services within these programs can help you decide if special arrangements would be more appropriate.

In most cases, attempts are made to keep the child in regular school to avoid isolating him from the support of friends and familiar teachers. This also may prevent him from feeling the stigma of attending a "special school" or being "handicapped." When the child does require special needs, the issue should be discussed with him depending on his age, if it appears to be a concern for him.

If your recovering child will be able to return to regular classes, it may help to ask the teacher to send schoolwork through a classmate, tape record classes, or provide reading material and makeup work to help your child stay on the same level as the other students until he can return. A "buddy system" for schoolwork will also help and encourage a close supportive relationship with at least one of his peers.

Helping your child to schedule homework, playtime, and treatments may also assure that he can keep up with the class. Depending on how your child feels about school and friends, he may be tempted to "goof off" to be like "one of the guys," or he may be diligent in his studies. It is important to let your child have some control of his schedule, but he will benefit from your continued guidance.

If your child misses days of school, it is important for you to keep track of the reasons for the absences. An increase in the frequency of absences should be evaluated to determine a change in health status, or it may indicate stress at school.[29] Recording the reasons for absences on a calendar or in a notebook provides a quick reference. It has also been suggested that once a pattern of absence is established, it is difficult to change.[30] Once again, continue an open dialogue about school, friends and teachers. This offers the opportunity for your child to express any problems, whether they be academic or personal.

Absence from school decreases the benefits of socializing with other children and can hurt the child's grades as well as his opportunities for further education. A review of the benefits of attending school (as described in the table) may help your child to realize its importance or may initiate an open discussion about what is bothering him. It has been shown that the level of anxiety is reduced with regular attendance.[31] Teachers, physicians, parents and the child with a life-threatening illness can carefully plan together and decide appropriate homework assignments, makeup work, workload, physical activities and vocational planning.

MEDICAL TREATMENT IN SCHOOL

Another factor to consider if your child is returning to school is whether or not he needs ongoing medication. Special arrangements may be necessary to assure that he receives appropriate doses of medicine at the right times throughout the day. You will need to have the physician sign medical papers to allow the school nurse to give your child medicine. It may help for the doctor to write a detailed list of the medications, the times to give them, and possible side effects school personnel should be aware of. You may ask the doctor to include a special note describing any changes in the child's health or behavior that should prompt school personnel to phone the parent or doctor. This can be important because side effects of medications may be interpreted by others to be symptoms of the illness or injury.

You and your child's physician both should feel free to telephone the school nurse or doctor to inquire about your child. A periodic conference with those involved with your child at school may help provide information about how he is adapting, whether or not there are changes in the quality of his work or in his behavior or whether medications seem to affect him differently during the day (making him sleepy, for example).[32] These conferences may also help you to periodically remind school personnel to enforce the medication schedule. Some children would prefer to miss medications than to be excused from class to go to the nurse or suffer side effects. Remind the teacher that medications are scheduled at certain times to provide optimal treatment.

Illness affects many aspects of a child's life, but there are numerous ways parents can help their child. In the hospital, parents can begin by explaining, listening, and even playing with their child. As the primary source of support, a parent can establish coping methods that work best for the child. As the child's advocate, the parent can make sure the hospital staff is aware of the child's special needs as well as his personal way of coping.

When a child returns home, he often encounters new stresses. Clinic visits, future hospitalizations, and returning to school all require adaptation as the child works through new feelings about his body and senses how friends, teachers, and even family members may feel differently about him. While helping the child recover from or adapt to a life-threatening illness entails hard work, it can also offer parents a deeper and more rewarding relationship with their child. A smile on the child's face when he triumphs can make it all worthwhile.

Notes

1. American Academy of Pediatrics, Committee on Hospital Care, *Hospital Care of Children and Youth* (1986); J. Goldberger, "Issue-specific Play With Infants and Toddlers in Hospitals: Rationale and Intervention," *Children's Health Care* 16 (Winter 1988): 134–41.

2. *Ibid.*, 135.

3. W. R. McWhirter and J. P. Masel, *Pediatric Oncology: An Illustrated Introduction* (Sydney: Williams & Wilkens and Associates, 1987), 67.

4. M. Gibbons and H. Boren, "Stress Reduction: A Spectrum of Strategies in Pediatric Oncology Nursing," *Nursing Clinics of North America* 20 (March 1985): 83–103.

5. C. Eiser, *The Psychology of Childhood Illness* (New York: Springer-Verlag, 1985), 55.

6. S. Maul-Mellot and J. Adams, *Childhood Cancer: A Nursing Overview* (Boston: Jones and Bartless Publishers, 1987), 31.

7. B. Riegel and D. Ehrenreich, *Psychological Aspects of Critical Care Nursing* (Rockville, Md.: Aspen Publishers, 1989), 265.

8. *The Merriam-Webster Dictionary* (New York: Pocket Books, 1974).

9. M. D. Pass and C. M. Pass, "Anticipatory Guidance for Parents of Hospitalized Children," *Journal of Pediatric Nursing* 2 (August 1987): 250–58.

10. D. B. Pruitt and M. Strickland, "Psychological Factors Affecting Children's Response to Medical Procedures: A Guide for Clinicians," *Psychiatric Medicine* 5 (1987): 206.

11. *Ibid.*, 203.

12. Goldberger, 139–140.

13. C. L. Betz and E. C. Poster, "Children's Concept of Death: Implications for Pediatric Practice," *Nursing Clinics of North America* 19 (June 1984): 341–49.

14. Betz, 344.

15. Betz, 346.

16. N. Hobbs and J. M. Perrin, eds. *Issues in the Care of Children With Chronic Illness* (San Francisco: Jossey-Bass 1985), 700.

17. M. A. Chesler and O. A. Barbarin, *Childhood Cancer and the Family: Meeting the Challenge of Stress and Support* (New York: Brunner/Mazel, 1987), 235.

18. M. M. Silverman and D. S. Katz, "Preventing Mental Health Problems," in R. E. K. Stein, *Caring for Children with Chronic Illness: Issues and Strategies* (1989): 213–229.

19. N. Hobbs, J. M. Perrin and H. T. Ireys, eds. *Chronically Ill Children and Their Families* (San Francisco: Jossey-Bass, 1985).

20. Eiser, 62.

21. D. W. Adams and E. J. Deveau, *Coping with Childhood Cancer: Where Do We Go from Here?* (Reston, Va.: Reston Publishing Company, 1984), 35.

22. S. Friedman and R. Hoekelman, *Behavioral Pediatrics: Psychosocial Aspects of Child Health Care* (New York: McGraw Hill, 1980), 202.

23. M. Weitzman, "School and Peer Relations," *Pediatric Clinics of North America* 31 (February 1984): 59–69.

24. Association for the Care of Children's Health, *Preparing Your Child for Repeated or Extended Hospitalizations* (1987).

25. Weitzman, 67.

26. Hobbs and Perrin, 710.

27. J. Van Eys, ed., *Children with Cancer: Mainstreaming and Integration* (New York: Spectrum Publications, 1982), 95.

28. I. D. Bullard and J. T. Dohnal, "The Community Deals with the Child Who Has a Handicap, *Chronic Nursing Clinics of North America* 19 (June, 1984): 309–318.

29. Friedman and Hoekelman, 202–204.

30. S. Lansky, "Management of Stressful Periods in Childhood Cancer," *Pediatric Clinics of North America* 32 (85):625–31.

31. Friedman and Hoekelman, 202–204.

32. Ross and Diserens, "Evaluations of a Symposium for Educators of Children with Cancer," *Journal of Psychosocial Oncology* 7 (1989): 159–178.

5

WHEN YOUR CHILD NEEDS INTENSIVE CARE

UNDERSTANDING THE STRESSES OF INTENSIVE CARE

For whatever reason your child requires intensive care, it can be a very frightening and emotionally draining experience. As the word "intensive" implies, your child will be under very close supervision and probably will receive many types of medical support to ensure that his body functions and recovers properly. During this intensive phase of hospitalization, you may feel even more alienated and unsure about your part in your child's care. Many of the suggestions offered in Chapter 3 may still apply to your child if intensive care becomes necessary. This new and frightening experience requires even more support and communication on your part. There are several ways you can help, depending on your child's physical status and extent of illness. Intensive care can be stressful for you both, but understanding some of the special stresses he may encounter can help you feel more confident and secure about interacting with him even when he is attached to specialized medical equipment.

ADMISSION INTO THE INTENSIVE CARE UNIT

The first stressful phase of intensive care may be the admission process. Depending on how your child is feeling, his awareness of the surroundings, and feelings of support from others, this new environment can be very overwhelming with noisy machines, new faces, strange equipment and intimidating procedures. He may have a sense of "unreality," as so much is happening at one time and he has little control.[1] In addition, parents may not be permitted to stay with the child during diagnostic or stabilizing procedures.

If you are not permitted to be with your child during admission, you might become fearful, confused and even angry. These are normal feelings that result from being denied the opportunity to be together at a time when you both need each other so much. Health professionals anticipate and understand these feelings. Some intensive care units have more liberal visitation policies than others, but rules vary and are ultimately determined by the health status of patients in each unit. Even though you cannot help feeling resentful, you should be aware of the reasons why you cannot be with your child. There may be several reasons for restricting your visitation:

1. Your child may become too excited, and this may cause his body undue stress.
2. Your child's body needs to rest in order to recover properly.
3. Procedures need to be done (especially on admission) and there is simply not enough room for you at the bedside.
4. The medical staff may want to protect you from getting upset at seeing a procedure and thus upsetting your child.
5. The medical staff might limit visitation to minimize noise, activity or chance of infection for all patients.
6. The staff might feel that your child would cooperate better if you were not there as his "protector."

Even though you may understand the reasons for limited visitation, your heart still tells you to be with your child. If for some reason you are not aware of your child's admission to the intensive care unit, or cannot be at the hospital, further feelings of anger, frustration and guilt will make it difficult for you to accept limited visits. Chapter 6 provides additional information about acknowledging your emotions in order to help yourself cope with different situations. This in turn will help you to communicate with the health team and thus be less tense when with your child.

There are several things that may help you during the time you are separated from your child. First, be assertive but calm and tactful when requesting information about your child, however, do not distract the health team when they are busy attending to him. It is particularly important to keep this in mind when you call and are put on hold for a long time!

If you feel comfortable being present during a procedure, and *you* feel your child will be more cooperative, tell his nurse or doctor that you think he will benefit from your presence. At other times, if your child's health status changes, you may need to wait outside while they attend to your child. The health care team will meet with you when they have information to provide. Remember, however, that not all restrictions on visits mean something is wrong! The physicians may simply be removing equipment or changing your child's treatment and assessing his response.

Most intensive care units encourage you to telephone at any time for a report. If you are awake at 3:00 A.M. and are wondering about your child, do not be afraid to call if you will sleep better knowing he is sleeping. (Remember, you will not be awakening the nurses.) This also applies if your work schedule forces you to call only at certain times, or if you are out and are afraid the hospital might try to reach you.

It might help to speak with other parents, perhaps in the parents' lounge, to see if they have suggestions about getting information or the best time to call. They may also have suggestions about how they cope themselves. You can also meet with a social worker or clergy member who can offer support by listening and comforting. Even with the support of others, you may feel depressed, angry or simply numb and may forget the information given to you. As stated before, don't be afraid to ask the same questions several times, or to ask for them to be more clearly explained. Stress makes it difficult to concentrate. In time, these feelings will subside as you become familiar with routines and equipment and understand expectations for your child's recovery process.

Just as you feel many emotions (or you may be too overwhelmed to feel them at all), your child may be feeling the same way. When you do get to see your child, it helps to remain calm, supportive and assuring. Explain why you cannot be with him all the time and acknowledge his feelings. Talking slowly and softly helps to promote a more secure atmosphere. When doctors or nurses are present, address them by name so your child can become familiar with them. If your child is unconscious, whether from the illness or anesthesia, do not be shy about talking to him. Talk as though he can hear you, reassuring him that you are there, that you love him and that he is getting help to get better. Touching your child, softly stroking an arm, brushing his hair back, or holding hands are comforting measures whether your child is awake or not. When your child is awake, request that the nurses and doctors speak directly to him, particularly when explaining various treatments or procedures. If you need information, request a conference with the medical team, or ask at the bedside, but relay the information to your child in terms that he can understand. This promotes less fear of the unknown and helps your child to feel a little more comfortable about the experience. It is important to be honest when answering your child's questions.

DEPRIVED SLEEP

Another aspect of intensive care is frequent interruption during sleep. Necessary procedures and medications that require schedules to promote optimal care may often mean waking your child. For this reason, if you visit your child when he is asleep, it may be best to allow him to remain asleep. If your visits are very limited, or you have been unable to see him for a while, ask how much sleep he has had to determine whether it would be alright to awaken him. Sometimes it is beneficial to awaken your child to reassure him of your support, especially if you will not be back for a while. Ask for assistance from the nurse if you are not sure what would be best.

The interruptions that awaken your child are often unpleasant in nature, and this contributes feelings of frustration and lack of control. When your child is awake, he may be more cranky, more apt to act out or more quiet than usual. Any of these behaviors can be normal reactions and are understood by health care professionals. Just as adults are more apt to become angry or irritable when tired, your child's behavior may simply indicate that he wants to rest. This may be his way of coping with the situation and his body's attempt to get better. Supporting your child's feelings reassures him that he is not being "bad."

CONFUSION ABOUT TIME AND PLACE

Patients in the intensive care unit may become confused about the time of day. This is due in part to the fact that intensive care units use constant lighting to observe the patients around the clock. Some units attempt to dim the lights at night to help promote the feeling of nighttime, and this can help to ease your child into restful sleep. The passage of time also is difficult to judge, so it may be helpful to provide a watch or calendar. Even watching favorite television shows can help the child gauge time. Holiday decorations can be cheerful but can also be reminders of being away from home at a special time. Special activities such as making his own decorations may help the child's morale.

If your child has been sedated, has had an operation or was unconscious when admitted to the intensive care unit, he will not know where he is upon awakening. Repeated explanations will probably be necessary to reassure him about what is happening and why and to make him comfortable with various types of equipment. You can request an overview of the unit (if it has not already been provided) so that you will be more informed and in turn can explain to your child. You may be surprised, however, to find that your child has no memory of the experience after leaving intensive care. Forgetting painful events may be a coping response, or he simply may not have been aware of what was happening.

NOISE

One obvious source of stress in intensive care is the continuous noise from machines or people talking and moving about. Everyone has a different sensitivity to sounds, and some children are more bothered by noise than others. Though there is little parents can do to reduce noise, helping your child to develop a way to cope may help.

If noise appears to be bothering him, ask if you can draw a curtain if one is available. Sometimes a battery-operated radio or headset helps to eliminate the noise from machines, but these must be approved by the medical team. If the radio is permitted, even though it is a source of noise, it is one your child has some control over. It also serves as a form of entertainment and distraction. Also, if people are talking too loudly, never hesitate to simply say, "My child is a little agitated, could you please speak a little softer?"

LACK OF PRIVACY

Children in intensive care units may experience a lack of privacy. The beds often are placed in open areas, which are necessary to accommodate large pieces of equipment and large numbers of medical personnel and to provide quick access in case of an emergency. Patients are visible to the staff, instead of being in closed rooms, to allow careful monitoring. While the intention is to ensure the best care for the patient, the exposure can cause feelings of embarrassment and lack of control, especially among children. The extent of embarrassment or sense of exposure may depend on the child's developmental level, awareness of the environment and perception of his body, as well as on which parts of the body are uncovered and examined.

If your child appears to be upset about this lack of privacy, discussions with nurses may make them aware of his needs; they may be able to provide a screen or curtain or may suggest ways how to help your child to cope. Your child may also become upset from seeing other seriously ill children or hearing them cry. It may be necessary to ask his nurse to explain procedures performed on other children, as a way of lessening his fears or misconceptions. Young children need a lot of support in understanding why other children are crying at certain times. Even in their own distress, they can be very empathetic toward others. On a positive note, however, your child may also learn new coping methods by watching these other children.

PHYSICAL STRESSES

Other obvious sources of stress for some children include restraints, which are necessary when a patient resists medical care and risks injuring himself. Traction, ventilator equipment used to help a patient to breathe, or various types of tubes required to support the patient's health also restrict a young child's movement and need for autonomy. Children and adolescents may initially require sedation to relax the body, maximize oxygen flow to the lungs or minimize trauma caused by resisting treatment.

You can offer significant support for your child by explaining why these treatments or procedures are necessary and by emphasizing, especially for younger children, that they are not punishment. While talking and playing with your child, take note if he fantasizes about the medical equipment. Toddlers or preschool children may imagine that tubes are snakes or that the machines are monsters or robots. Even older children who become confused from medications or become disoriented in the busy intensive care unit can have similar thoughts. You can assist health professionals by making them aware of these behaviors. With this information, they may adjust their plan of care or change the way they interact with the patient and thus maximize treatment. You might tape snapshots, pictures from siblings (or one your child has drawn) or other familiar items onto the equipment in view of your child (if approved by the medical staff). This may help to make the equipment less frightening.

A child in intensive care is subject to intense stress. Behavior may change as a result, and ongoing support may be necessary after leaving the intensive care unit, but remember that the purpose of intensive care is to provide the best care for your child when seriously ill. Support from parents and health care workers can help the child to cope and to emerge with a sense of accomplishment from overcoming new challenges.

POSSIBLE REACTIONS AND BEHAVIORS AND WAYS TO HELP YOUR CHILD

REACTIONS AND BEHAVIORS

The stress of intensive care can trigger behavior similar to that exhibited during general hospitalization. Children may have periodic nightmares or restless sleep, they may want a parent to sleep with them or they may seek a security object, such as a special blanket or stuffed animal. One study found that these behaviors disappeared two to four weeks after the child returned home, but that the child needed to discuss the hospitalization in detail.[2]

New behaviors may also develop and cannot always be anticipated. If your child was previously on another hospital floor and appeared to cope well, you may be suddenly surprised to see a different reaction to intensive care. He may act out, become withdrawn, blame you for the illness or injury, deny the illness or even show signs of grief. If your child feels out of control, fears death, or is having difficulty accepting the many new painful procedures, he may act differently than you have seen before. Several possible behaviors include:[3]

- An unwillingness to talk about the illness
- Inappropriate attempts to direct his own treatment
- Lack of cooperation with limits on activities
- Frequent questions about care—i.e., "What was my temperature?"
- Withdrawal from family members
- Loss of trust in parents or care givers
- Expressing feelings of worthlessness or insecurity
- Frequent crying
- Frequent yelling or hitting
- Refusal to participate in care
- Denying changes in his body (scars, burns, etc.)

Some children may rely on coping strategies that have helped in the past, and parents can encourage these to help their child adapt to the new environment. Parents can also inform the health care team about these coping strategies so they can also promote them when the parents are not able to be with the child.

For some children, behaviors can be based on their interpretation of what is happening to specific body parts. Children who require transplants or major surgery on an organ may have preconceived ideas about that organ. For example, young children may know the heart as a symbol of love and may become confused as to why it needs repair. They need to be shown what the actual heart looks like, how it functions and why it is being "fixed" or replaced.[4] Children having transplants also need to understand the transplant process and need assurance that they will receive a new, healthier organ that will make them better. Children may be confused, however, when they feel pain after the surgery—after having been told that they were going to feel better. It is therefore essential to teach each child what to expect and how the pain will be relieved. This will help to maintain trust among parents, health care providers and the child.

Another aspect of intensive care that parents may have difficulty discussing with their child is the fear of death. If your child has been ill and suddenly requires intensive care, his fears about death may surface. These fears are different for everyone, depending on age and previous experiences with serious illness. Parents who experienced a relative dying in intensive care are more likely to associate intensive care with death, and thus have more fear of their own child dying. Anxiety about death will also differ for families of children who knew intensive care would be required following surgery rather than those requiring it from complications from the surgery or illness. The potential for death is also perceived differently when a child is placed in intensive care as a result of physical trauma such as a fall or car accident. The sudden change of having a healthy child to one requiring advanced health care is a shock, maybe compounded by feelings of guilt, and perceptions of the experience may then be more overwhelming and fearful.

Any concerns about the possibility of death or of future intensive care, even concerns that seem trivial to the parents or the child, should be brought to the attention of a doctor, nurse, social worker or other member of the health team in order to assure an accurate understanding of the prognosis and what it entails for the future. Thus the family and child can better prepare themselves, avoid misconceptions and lessen anxiety about the unknown.

SUGGESTIONS FOR HELPING YOUR CHILD IN INTENSIVE CARE

Any of these behaviors may be surprising and hard to accept at first. It is important to remember, however, that your child is unsure how to act at this time and still needs your guidance. If your child is acting out, remain loving but firm in your response to his actions. Perhaps ask the nurses how they have been helping your child during these difficult times. They may be able to lend proven advice. Remembering that cooperation is vital to his health may help you be stern in those times you may feel guilty about disciplining him when he is so ill. Consistency in your response also demonstrates that some things have not changed. You may learn to be flexible with changes in his condition, degree of responsiveness and varying emotions. It can help to remember that your child will continually test your willpower in managing his behavior.

It may also help to establish a routine when you are visiting. If you wish, ask if you can give your child a bath, perhaps at a set time each day. This will give you time together—time to talk and to touch, and time for security. If certain treatments or procedures are scheduled, and you feel able, ask if you can participate in some way, perhaps by passing non-sterile equipment to the nurse, helping your child with coping techniques such as imagery or focusing, or simply holding hands.

Sometimes children in intensive care require special exercises to maintain muscle tone when they are bedridden. This is another opportunity to learn about your child's care and perhaps to participate. When a nurse is available to teach you, simply ask if there is anything you can learn to do. If you are not comfortable with performing these new tasks, it is best not to force it, as you may feel awkward and in turn may convey your tension or anxiety to your child. Initially you may be a little anxious, but anxiety can be overcome with practice. Follow your feelings and guidance from the staff on the unit. There may come a time when it will be necessary for you to learn these routines, as you and your child prepare for discharge from the hospital.

If your child is unable to speak but is alert, you can help him establish a communication system. Depending on his age and his ability to write or to move his body, you may be able to help him communicate through writing notes, blinking his eyes, counting fingers, tapping fingers, or raising his right or left arm or hand for "yes" and "no."

You are the person most attuned to your child's responses, and you will be better at interpreting his body language or attempts at communication. The child who is unable to speak has an added frustration that contributes to feelings of loss of control. Helping him to communicate can significantly boost his morale as well as provide valuable information to the health professionals about his condition.

Parents can also help the health care team assess whether or not their child is in pain when he is unable to speak. Nurses and physicians are experienced in assessing pain in children, but parents are more aware of subtle changes in their child's behavior. This is especially true for younger children, who cannot always verbally express when they are in pain.

Another way you can help your child is to allow him to do things for himself such as wash his own face, brush his teeth, or use a radio and earphones.

If your child must eat in a special way, ask if you can learn to feed him. If you are comfortable with feeding, bathing, or helping with certain exercises, these can be wonderful opportunities to interact with your child. The nurses or doctors will explain when you are not able to help but will appreciate your willingness to participate.

Listed on page 88 are several suggestions for helping your child during his stay in intensive care. Knowing his temperament and capabilities, along with advice from his nurse or physician, you can help decide which suggestions to try.[5]

REMEMBERING PLAY

Sometimes children need to be reassured that it is okay to play when they are physically able. You may need to initiate play to show your

SUGGESTIONS FOR HELPING THE CHILD IN INTENSIVE CARE

Reassure your child about what he is able to do

Provide time for play therapy

Encourage your child to cooperate when receiving regular care, medications, treatments and therapies

Continue his regular bedtime rituals when possible

Bring a toy or a favorite item from home

Provide opportunities for him to discuss his feelings and the purposes for treatments or procedures, how they are done, and how they will benefit him (such as getting out of the intensive care unit)

If positive reinforcement does not promote cooperation, be consistent about discipline

Answer questions honestly

Encourage appropriate coping strategies

Be observant of your child's responses

Inform the nurse or doctor of any changes

Allow your child choices whenever possible

Encourage creative activities

Change the environment to provide some stimulation

child that he is able to do certain things, but it is important not to force him if he is not ready. Offer books, tapes, cards, or even games if he is up to it. Stuffed animals for young children can provide a secure, familiar object to clutch and to exercise fingers, hands and arms and stimulate the eyes. As your child's condition improves, see if it is possible for creative play such as painting, cutting up magazines to make a collage or making pictures with glitter. This type of activity may be particularly helpful if your child becomes aggressive or frustrated from being in an isolated environment.[6] For younger children, fantasy play such as having a picnic or tea party, or role-playing, can allow them to "experiment more freely with feelings and situations."[7] It has been shown that play can positively influence the child's attitude about his environment.[8]

However frustrating, it is important to remember why there may be times you will not be able to visit your child in intensive care. The staff's priorities are to stabilize your child's health, perform necessary treatments and procedures and allow him time to rest. It is also difficult not to feel guilty if you are unable to be at your child's side because of other commitments, but you may have other siblings to take care of, you may need to work to pay medical bills, or you may simply need a break. Talking with the staff, the social worker, and friends or relatives may help to provide solutions.

In addition to concerns about being with your child, you might also worry about the new stresses placed upon him in intensive care. Depending on the circumstances surrounding his admission, the amount of time he has had to prepare and his developmental level, your child might react in various ways. Trying to respond to his needs, the change in his physical status, new schedules, and new faces makes it a tough time for you as the parent. Remember that your child may be sensitive to your reactions as he seeks reassurance from you about what is happening. Learning about the new things can enable you to help him work through his feelings and fears. Work at your own pace so that you are comfortable with what you are learning, and perhaps you will feel more secure when interacting with your child.

Notes

1. B. Riesel and D. Ehrenreich, *Psychological Aspects of Critical Care Nursing* (Rockville, Md.: Aspen Publishers, 1989), 17, n. 23.

2. H. P. Gabriel and D. A. Danilowicz, "Open-Heart Surgery for Congenital Heart Disease: Minimizing Adverse Psychological Sequelae in Families Facing Major High-Risk Surgery," in A. E. Christ and K. Flomenhaft, eds., *Psychosocial Family Interventions in Chronic Pediatric Illness* (New York: Plenum Press, 1982), 107.

3. Riegel and Ehrenreich, 17–23.

4. Gabriel and Danilowicz, 107.

5. M. Shandor Miles and M. C. Carter, "Coping Strategies Used By Parents During Their Child's Hospitalization in an Intensive Care Unit," *Child Health Care* 14 (Summer 1985): 14–21.

6. S. Gottlieb and S. Portney, "The Role of Play in a Pediatric Bone Marrow Transplantation Unit," *Children's Health Care* 16 (Winter 1988): 161–65.

7. Gottlieb and Portney, p. 187.

8. S. O'Connell, "Recreation Therapy: Reducing the Effects of Isolation for the Patient in the Protected Environment," *Children's Health Care* 12 (1984): 118–21; J. Pearson et al., "Pediatric Intensive Care Unit Patients: Effects of Play Intervention on Behavior," *Critical Care Medicine* 8 (1980): 64–67.

6

PARENTING

INTERPERSONAL STRESS

Being a parent is one of life's most unique and rewarding experiences. Parents and children contribute to each other's development and share memorable and emotional times. The pain and frustration of a life-threatening illness can overshadow the joys of raising a child as well as the pleasures a parent and child can share. Many concerns over health care, finances and healthy siblings, as well as the ill child can dramatically change family priorities.

By acknowledging that relationships will probably change and can add to stress, this may help parents to work through the experience.

The following information covers issues faced by the parent and suggests ways a parent might handle them. Specific courses of action are best decided on among those closest to the family and the child's own health care team.

YOU AND THE MEDICAL STAFF: FEELING IN CONTROL

Many stresses can affect how you feel about your child's illness and treatment. Some parents feel better when they "leave everything" to the health professionals. Others want to be actively involved with the child's care. Being involved allows you to feel more in control and more informed yet can in itself be a source of stress. Getting to know the medical staff and understanding their expectations can help you feel more confident in the course of treatment. This includes feeling more in control over the care your child receives. Dissatisfaction with health care has been found to be associated with more specialized care and advanced technology. A parent's lack of understanding of care can lead to unrealistic expectations for a child's treatment and recovery. In addition, some parents may feel the medical staff tends to overlook the child's emotional needs and less time is available for family consultations. When parents' expectations are not met, frustration and lack of communication can compound the feelings of lack of control and helplessness.

Dr. Raymond Mulhern of St. Jude's Children's Hospital in Memphis, Tennessee emphasizes that parents should not feel intimidated or rushed when they need to know information.[1] Some parents feel better learning about medications, the disease process or various procedures in great detail. If the health professionals seem rushed, wait for a quieter moment, but be sure to make your needs known before they leave the room. If it appears there is no time, simply say "I have a question when you have a moment." Write the question down, and remind them as soon as you see them again. It is part of their job to explain your child's condition. After all, it is safer and less confusing for you and your child to ask questions than to assume the wrong thing. Parents can also help prevent the kind of misunderstandings that can happen on a busy floor filled with many professionals working together. The staff may be able to anticipate some of your concerns, but they need to be made aware of issues that are important to you at any given time.

Two professors of nursing, S. E. Thorne and C. A. Robinson, have suggested three distinct stages that family members go through when dealing with health professionals caring for their child, particularly when the illness is chronic or requires intermittent or extended hospitalization. As in any relationship, understanding and acceptance of others takes time. The stages are:

Naive Trusting:
Family members may initially assume that care will be a cooperative effort between the family and the health care team and that decisions will be made together. They may assume that the professionals' view of what is best for the child will be the same as the family's. Differences arise as members of the health care team continue to focus on the illness while the family tries to minimize the effects of the illness in an effort to normalize the child's life.

Disenchantment:
If there is a lack of understanding between the health care team and the child and family, the family may become dissatisfied with the care. This may result in negative attitudes toward health care providers and toward hospital policies and routines. Frustration and fear may ultimately be expressed as anger, especially when the family attempts to obtain information or change aspects of care.

Guarded Alliance:
As continuous care for the child becomes necessary, the family may begin to reestablish a sense of trust with members of the health care team by acknowledging both the strengths and limitations of specific care providers. Family members may begin to feel more comfortable in pursuing information. They may also become more involved in promoting positive experiences for the child. Frustrations may continue (such as periods of having to wait or not knowing what to ask),

but there will be a better understanding of the "values and priorities underlying both the policies of the system and the behaviors of the individual professionals so that many situations [can] be anticipated and manipulated."[2]

These stages demonstrate how feelings may change over the course of treatment and why it is essential to know the health care team in order for you to feel comfortable with your child's treatment. Some families may progress through these stages, while others may remain either satisfied or dissatisfied with care. Each child's treatment is unique, and experiences will vary for each family member and health professional. To some extent, you can help determine how positive the experience will be by openly communicating with those involved in your child's care.

In order to feel comfortable in communicating information to your child and reinforcing the necessity of medications and procedures, you must trust those people treating your child. If you are unsure of the reasons for medications, treatments or procedures, simply ask and if necessary, ask again, then relay that information to your child if you feel that he does not understand. If after receiving information you still do not feel the procedure or medication is necessary, or if it contradicts what you have been told before, request a conference with the physician responsible for treating your child so that you can voice your concerns.

Sometimes parents feel the need to seek second opinions, even from untrained and uninformed sources who offer unproven methods of treatment.[3] This can be very dangerous to the vulnerable parent who will do almost anything in hope of finding a cure or a way to improve his child's health. Once again, communication with the physician and health care workers is essential in providing the best care for your child.

Obtaining a second opinion can be difficult while your child is in the hospital. If you truly question your child's treatment, discuss your concerns with someone you trust, perhaps a nurse or social worker. They may be able to refer you to another physician specializing in your child's illness. There may be a physicians' list or information number you can obtain from the hospital or community organization so you can ask questions and feel reassured. Each hospital has an ethics committee or a patient advocacy group. Call the hospital's general information number to locate them. For cancer patients, the Office of Cancer Communications at the National Cancer Institute in Bethesda, Maryland provides a physician search and a list of NCI-sponsored protocols of treatment (listed in Appendix A).

It is important to feel that your child is receiving appropriate care. It is also important to remember, however, that physicians are always seeking better ways of treating life-threatening illnesses, and they ultimately hope to find a cure. This often involves ongoing research, with different methods of treatment, and treatment may vary from hospital to hospital. Your child's physician is the first person you should consult so that you can understand his reasons for procedures and medications. Then you will have as much information as possible, which will be helpful if you do seek assistance from others. Before signing consent forms, be sure you are comfortable with the information offered to you. Things to consider include:[4]

- Is the treatment experimental?
- What are other treatment options, if any?
- What are the risks and benefits of the proposed treatment?
- What are the possible short-term side effects?
- What are the possible long-term side effects?

Understanding these aspects of treatment will allow you to make a more informed decision. It is also the physician's obligation to make sure you are aware of them.

If your child is in a teaching hospital, most of which are affiliated with a university, he will probably be seen by many doctors in different levels of training. You may feel reassured by the fact that several people are involved in your child's care and that they share information and opinions. On the other hand, your child will be forced to interact with more people, and you might be asked to repeat his medical history several times. The chart on page 97 explains the hierarchy of physicians in a hospital.[5]

While going to the "top" doctor may help to resolve difficulties with other physicians on the floor, it may be more helpful to first communicate your concerns to the physician most directly involved with your child's care. Speaking with your child's nurse or social worker may also provide more information, as well as support, if you ultimately need to speak with the attending physician or chief resident.

Differences of opinion may also occur between parents and other health care workers, such as nurses or respiratory or physical therapists. Once again, direct communication with medical staff will allow them to understand why you are upset and to explain the way they are working. In some cases, they may not be aware of special circumstances of your child's condition. If, after the discussion, the situation does not improve, you may communicate your concerns to a professional you trust or go to the supervisor of the person you are having difficulties with.

As discussed in Chapter 1, it is important that you feel comfortable with and trust those caring for your child. There will be less stress, and

Attending physician:	An experienced doctor who is ultimately responsible for the daily care of all patients on the unit, overseeing other doctors' orders and treatment plans
Chief resident:	A doctor who has served several years as a resident or fellow and has developed specialized skills in his area of interest
Fellow:	A doctor who decides to obtain more specialized training, continuing with two or three additional years past residency
Resident:	A doctor who has usually completed one year as an intern and continues with specialty training for two to four years
Intern:	A doctor who has graduated medical school and is beginning to train in a specialty such as pediatrics, surgery or internal medicine
Medical student:	A person in his or her seventh or eighth year of medical school who is in training on the patient floor

you will be less apt to feel guilty about not having taken an active role if your child's health status changes. You are best suited to act as your child's advocate and to see that your family's needs are met by the staff.

STRESS AND COPING

GENERAL FAMILY ISSUES

When illness or injury strikes a child, stress levels for parents increase as they try to meet the many new demands placed on their child and family. You may find that you have taken on a new role as the family "advocate" to assure that all needs are being met. You may feel that you give so much, only to feel overwhelmed and misunderstood at times. The illness or injury has obvious effects on your child. But with so many changes and added responsibilities, how are you and the rest of the family affected?

Each family functions in a unique way, with its own schedule of activities that may be consistent or vary from day to day. Illness will therefore influence each family differently, depending on the following factors:[6]

- The age of the child when illness or injury first occurs
- The course of the illness or injury, i.e., is it stable or are there periods of increased severity?
- Does the prognosis offer an improvement or decline in health status?
- The illness's effect on the child's ability to move around, i.e., can the child do self-care, be independent?
- The illness's effect on the child's intellectual abilities
- Predictability of care, i.e., can there be unexpected hospitalizations? Are there routine treatment schedules?
- Visible manifestations of the illness, i.e., what symptoms of the illness are obvious, what side effects of treatments or medications are easily seen?

The more factors negatively affecting your child and family, the more support and assistance you will need. When it is possible, you should consider accepting assistance to minimize stress levels and promote a healthier environment for everyone. This can be very difficult for a family that has been independent and takes pride in helping others. It may help to remember that by accepting support (which comes in many ways and will be discussed later), you are able to be more actively involved with your child and will remain emotionally, perhaps physically, stronger to be the family advocate.

PERSONAL STRESS

Parents (and perhaps children) may go through several emotional stages during the course of a child's illness, particularly when it is chronic.[7] They are:

1. Shock, disbelief or bewilderment
2. Fear, frustration, anger and resentment
3. Sadness: mourning the loss of your healthy child
4. Acceptance: asking questions and planning
5. Anger
6. Reacceptance, or mourning if the child dies

When a parent first learns about his child's illness or injury, he may deny that it is actually happening, or he may feel emotionally numb.

Temporary denial can be a healthy coping strategy if it balances the parent's emotions and gives him time to prepare for what lies ahead. As long as the denial does not impede the child's treatment, health professionals will understand the reaction. They are aware that sudden changes that come with hospitalization—new faces, the need to absorb new information quickly—may make the experience seem like a dream. Sometimes parents cannot remember information that has been given to them, and this can be a normal response to the stress. Some parents may convince themselves that their child "will recover despite indications to the contrary, while other [parents] fear the worst despite hopeful signs."[8] When you are able to accept the illness, it is important for your child to also work through his emotions and grasp the reality of the situation.

As reality does set in, you may become angry at the unfairness of the illness or injury, and this anger can be directed toward yourself, others and even subconsciously toward your child. The stress may leave you tired and irritable and you may snap at others more easily. You may also find yourself resenting healthy children or even the professionals who offer less than what you had hoped. As the emotional roller coaster continues, you may begin to feel guilty about *these* feelings. You may find yourself crying easily, having trouble sleeping and even having the urge to escape all of the problems. These are normal responses to the stress and frustration of your child's serious illness or injury.

As treatment or rehabilitation progresses, you may begin to feel sad, perhaps depressed, at the circumstances your family has been forced to endure. Added responsibilities, lost opportunities, and a changed family life may be overwhelming, especially if you are unsure where to find support.

After some time, you may begin to accept these changes as new family roles and responsibilities establish themselves. It has been stated that "most parents need time to adjust privately to the reality of their child's illness before they can deal with it in public."[9] Tolerance is built over time as experiences are absorbed and dealt with and a more stable life becomes possible. As you begin to accept the experience, you may find it easier to ask for support from others. If there are changes in the illness or rehabilitation—unexpected setbacks, exacerbations of the illness or new health problems—you and your child may have to confront loss of control and anger all over again. Finally, you may reach the last stage of acceptance, when you have established coping methods, setbacks are dealt with and supported, and life has once again settled into some sort of a routine. If your child's health status has instead declined and death is imminent, you may begin to be able to mourn.

Once again, each family is unique and it is impossible to predict how each member will or should react. You as a parent can cope in several ways: you can learn about the illness to minimize your anxiety and confusion, plan ways to normalize everyone's life as much as possible, and seek support from others.

It is important for you to acknowledge stress and to be aware of your own limitations. Your child will not benefit if you become overwhelmed and stressed to the point that your own physical or emotional health is endangered. Acknowledging stresses allows you to cope directly with them, and in turn lets you provide the most effective support for your ill child and family. Just as there are many variables that affect your hospitalized child, there are several variables that can affect your own stress level.

When a child is first diagnosed or injured, "parents are often confused, vulnerable and have little chance to establish coping strategies . . . and feel more comfortable and in control by learning and knowing about the illness itself." [10] By learning about the illness, you can begin to anticipate what will happen next and be able to plan. Learning about the illness, however, can be a stressful process in itself. Many feelings and emotions that occur as a result of having a seriously ill child are absolutely normal. Guilt, loss of confidence in being a good parent, anger, frustration, impatience, loss of religious faith, helplessness, isolation, fear, resentment, depression and grief are a few of the emotions you can experience at any given time. [11] You may be surprised to learn that health professionals are sympathetic to such emotions and may experience them themselves in their work with sick children.

You may sometimes feel unable to cooperate and may become overprotective about your child. You may suddenly find yourself angry at the doctors, and you may even yell. This anger can be a result of not wanting to accept the diagnosis or being angry at not being able to do more for your child.

If you feel these emotions surfacing, keep in mind that you do not want to upset your child or disrupt his relationship with his health care providers. The health professionals may offer suggestions to help you cope. You may interpret their comments as criticisms of you as a parent, but in most cases the professionals are simply offering advice that has been helpful to other parents. Remembering two things may help to redirect your anger. First, know that everyone is concerned with the child's best interest, and second, you are recognized as the most significant support for your child. Talking with someone you trust or with other parents may help. With greater understanding of the disease or injury, it may become easier to differentiate the trivial complaints from the significant ones. This helps you more effectively manage your child's care by communicating your thoughts and concerns in a constructive way.

YOU AND YOUR PARTNER

As a result of these roller-coaster emotions, you and your partner may find that your relationship is strained. Arguments can arise over even trivial matters when tensions are high. Even bigger arguments might erupt during critical stages of treatment, when the child returns home, or when a setback occurs.

Most parents do not want or need these conflicts but are unsure how to handle them. Understanding some of the reasons for the stress that might trigger a fight may help to restore communication between parents or partners. Marriage counseling has helped many to communicate and learn to cope with stress. Some parents find it difficult to find time for counseling amid the child's hospitalizations, new emotional needs and added family responsibilities. But enabling parents or partners to better work together will help support the child and perhaps make him feel more secure. It is difficult for some seriously ill children not to blame themselves when their parents are upset, fight or separate during or shortly after the illness or injury.

Some difficulties commonly experienced by parents or partners with an ill child are described below. These do not necessarily create marital difficulties in all families nor can they always be avoided in healthy relationships. Awareness of these factors can provide a foundation for understanding and communication between partners during times of disagreement.[12]

Recent research has shown, however, that illness may not always result in strained relationships.[13] Some spouses or partners may actually grow closer together as they support one another, openly express needs and communicate more. Focusing on each other's strengths also helps to maintain support, helps to determine what each partner can do to maximize family coping and promotes a positive environment that encourages hope rather than despair.

PARENTING ISSUES

Some parents also are concerned about "parenting issues," such as providing time for siblings, disciplining the ill child, providing medical care at home after the child is dismissed from the hospital. Caring for the ill child takes a lot of time, including time away from the rest of the family. Parental roles may change; for example, the father may have to assume

STRESSES THAT MAY AFFECT MARRIAGES OR PARTNERSHIPS

Some mothers or fathers begin to feel overburdened with the responsibilities of caring for the ill child.

Some mothers or fathers feel isolated as they work to meet financial needs but are away from the ill child.

Thoughts and feelings are not shared by one or both of the partners, and misconceptions develop from assuming the wrong thing.

One parent feels the partner is favoring the ill child over healthy siblings.

One parent feels the partner is avoiding the ill child and focusing on a healthy sibling.

Blame and criticism is offered instead of sympathy and understanding.

Problems from the past resurface and are focused upon instead of supporting the ill child and family.

One or both parents focus on the negative aspects of the illness or treatment instead of promoting positive times together.

One or both parents are frustrated by having limited time together, and by the fact that the child's needs take precedence over everyone else's.

One partner disagrees with or does not understand the other partner's coping strategies (such as reading, drinking, doing crafts).

more household chores while the mother is at the hospital with the child. Loss of employment by one parent who desires to be with the ill child may increase the financial burden. Less time together means fewer opportunities to talk *and* listen. Time spent together may be affected by fatigue and irritability. Siblings' needs must be addressed as well. Over all, the family may start to feel out of control and isolated.

With so many changes, needs and expectations, and fear of the unknown, how do family members cope and remain close? You may wonder how to divide responsibilities so that everyone has a fair share of work and how to arrange time for everyone to be together. Despite the disruptions in family life, many families find ways to adjust. Some have conquered the strongest odds and become a source of support for other families. Some have even initiated new legislation related to health care.

The following suggestions for coping are based on professional and parental recommendations.[14]

Be flexible whenever possible, alternating time with the ill child and household duties. Arrange sibling visits so everyone can have family time together.

Share decisions about treatments, household concerns or family matters. The illness provides enough surprises.

Support the personal growth of each family member.

Contact support groups or organizations that can benefit the child and family.

Share responsibilities for care of the ill child.

Share information about the illness, treatments, support groups, and prognosis.

Maintain normal activities whenever possible.

Do not take emotional outbursts of family members to be personal; consider current stresses.

Offer support, but accept it as well.

Make time for yourself, including an occasional "date" with your partner. Providing for your own needs will in time enable you to be more helpful to your child and family.

If problems seem to get out of hand or are difficult to resolve, seek help from others.

Talk with the physician about planning a family vacation when the ill child is physically able to travel.

While some of these suggestions seem to be common sense, they help to remind partners to communicate and support one another during times of stress. An emotionally stable and happy family reduces stress in the seriously ill child. Parents can also be strong role models for the child to learn successful coping methods.

CHANGES IN THE FAMILY

Hospitalization affects every family member's schedule to some degree. Parents must work out a schedule to provide time with the ill child, time with siblings, time to do family chores and take care of finances. When several people share these responsibilities, the physical and emotional burden is eased. This may create new problems, however, as conflicts may arise over who should do what, and when and how these tasks should be carried out. With so much change, family members may begin to feel like jugglers. You may find yourself thinking "Which hat should I wear today?"

Again, communication among family members is essential. By talking and listening, you will reduce the chance of one person feeling overburdened, left out or misunderstood. One way to enhance communication may be to sit down together and make schedules, providing for some flexibility when possible. Making a schedule gives each member of the family some feeling of control and a clear understanding of what is expected. The following is a sample schedule for a weekend while a child, Joe, is receiving a treatment at the hospital:

	FRIDAY	SATURDAY	SUNDAY
Mom	with Joe	home, then Joe	Sara's recital
Dad	working	with Joe	Sara's recital
Sara	school/dinner	ballet, Joe	Sara's recital
Uncle Bill			with Joe

This is of course a simplified version of scheduling at a time when a child may not be critically ill. It does, however, provide the foundation for a family to set up a system that will work for them. You can also maintain a communication board somewhere in the home, such as on the refrigerator or by the phone, where family members can check schedules or leave messages. This provides a back-up if schedules need to be rearranged or something unforeseen happens. If financially possible, an answering machine can also be useful.

Child care and household tasks become a big concern when parents need to work or be at the hospital with the ill child. A strong support system may become necessary, and may be difficult to initiate. Parents often do not want to burden family and friends with child care responsibility or the mundane tasks of household chores and grocery shopping. If you find that you need help in this area, however, do not be afraid to make your needs known. Some people are very willing to assist a family who has an ill child but may not be sure how to offer help. You may wish to approach close friends or family members who you feel may be comfortable helping you. If offers to help are made, simply state that some assistance will be very helpful and you will work out a schedule that will not be too inconvenient for them.

For example, you may say to a neighbor, "If you don't mind, could you please pick up some milk, bread and lunch meat for me when you go to the store. I'll walk over and get it when I get home from the hospital." You can also ask a relative to stay with or pick up the children one day each week. Establishing some sort of a routine is more comforting to younger children when it is possible. Additional information about siblings is provided in Chapter 7.

Social workers, health professionals, or local community organizations are available to contact when you need assistance with arranging child care or transportation. Additional support services and resources are listed in Appendix A. These resources are especially important to the single parent who may easily become overwhelmed and in turn may not be able to fully respond to all needs of his ill child. It is important for all families to let the health care team know when they need assistance so they can be directed to the appropriate resources.

DISCIPLINING THE ILL CHILD

One area of parental concern that may not always be addressed in the hospital is disciplining the ill child. Health issues take priority, and unless the child is very uncooperative or combative during hospitalization, the parent may not be concerned about punishment for bad behaviors. Research over the past few decades has shown, however, that lack of discipline is actually more confusing to the child, and behavior problems may result if his behavior is not properly guided.[15] In addition, poor cooperation during medical procedures or medications can hinder the recovery process and even endanger the child's health.

Part of the dilemma in guiding a child's behavior comes from the difficulty in distinguishing which behavior results from treatments, medications and fear and which is willful acting out (i.e., testing parents to see how much they can get away with).[16] Parents worry that their expectations may be too high or not appropriate, especially when the child regresses to earlier developmental behaviors to cope with stress. What if the child is really trying to cooperate, but is simply getting frustrated or does not understand? Won't discipline create more frustration? The hardest part of discipline in this situation is the parent's acceptance that it is needed.[17]

Unfortunately, no step-by-step directions are available for every situation. The first step in preventing negative behavior is to provide your child with opportunities for increased control, in addition to rewarding good behavior. But no child is perfect, so what happens when he *does* act out or does not cooperate? Previous experience with ill children has shown that setting limits provides security and establishes expectations that can be discussed and modified to suit each family's needs. It establishes routines and expectations at a time when illness creates confusion and uncertainty. It may help to remember that even healthy children need guidance, and too much freedom can frighten the child and make him feel insecure.[18] By continuing with previous methods of discipline, being understanding yet firm, you can make your child's life normal and stable to some extent. It also helps to establish guidance for behavior at school. In his own experience counseling families, Dr. Raymond Mulherm of St. Jude's Children's Hospital in Memphis, Tennessee has found that the second most frequent discipline problem occurs in school.[19] With continued discipline, siblings are also assured that the parent is not favoring the ill child. Seeing that some things have not changed will be reassuring to everyone in the family.

In considering what may cause behavior changes that can test a parent's patience, several factors associated with negative behaviors include: helplessness, boredom, hopelessness, fear, anger, side effects from medications and frustration from changes in life-style.

If behavior changes during stressful times in the course of the illness, tolerance and understanding are recommended as the best approach.[20] Praise your child when he does *not* revert to regressive behavior. At other times, when behavior is more defiant, gentle and consistent discipline to establish boundaries can prevent the behavior from developing into a pattern.[21] Offer examples of alternative, acceptable behavior to help your child understand what you expect from him. School-aged children may be more sensitive to what is socially acceptable, and may be more willing to comply. It may be helpful to offer creative outlets through play, sports or group activities. Some parents have found that removing privileges is the best method of discipline for the ill child when communication breaks down.

One technique used to calm children is to call "time out" when they misbehave. This method involves disciplining the child by seating him in a "time out" chair or corner for a certain amount of time. This allows him to regain control of his behavior and teaches him the consequences of bad behavior. *Explain what behavior will result in "time out"* and then be consistent and follow through by calmly placing your child where he cannot play or interact with others. Use a timer if it is available. Do not give your child warnings such as "the next time you do that I'll put you in time out!"; if you do, he will probably begin to test you to see how far the behavior can go. Explain that additional punishment will result if he does not comply—that he will lose privileges or be spanked. This can be an effective form of discipline when it is used consistently.

Another technique that is sometimes used in hospitals when a child is uncooperative is the "contract" for good behavior. The main purpose of the contract is to emphasize positive behavior. Roberta Babbitt, a behavior analyst and director of outpatient services for the Kennedy

Institute for Handicapped Children in Baltimore, Maryland emphasizes that the purpose of contracting is not necessarily getting your child to behave, but providing goals for him to achieve. A reward system must accompany the contract to motivate your child to behave well. On the following page is a sample contract for an eight year old hospitalized for a bone marrow transplant.

The contract should list what is expected of the child and why, when, where and how each activity or behavior should be done. Design a chart, calendar or diary that allows the child to place stickers or a mark when each activity or positive behavior occurs. A reward system should be mutually decided between the child and parent. Contracting emphasizes good behavior and sets goals for the child and purposely does not focus on negative behaviors. It is important, however, to also list punishments or consequences for failure to complete the contract. Set a time or date when the contract will be completed or reviewed for changes or updates.

Both the child and the parent (and health care providers if they are involved) should sign the contract to show their commitment and understanding of what is expected. In order for the contract to work, parents must enforce all consequences and be prompt with rewards.

Contracts have been established to improve compliance of children as young as two or three years old but have been found to be very helpful for adolescents as well. (Noncompliance, however, is more frequent among adolescents.) Contracting can contribute to the recovery process and can prevent the development of the behavioral problems that may result from the stress of illness or hospitalization.

Even if a contract is not established, rewarding good behavior through extra privileges, praise and hugs provides positive attention instead of concentrating on the negative aspects of the child's temperament.[22] Dr. Linda Dahlquist, of Ballor College of Medicine in Houston, Texas suggests that older children also react positively to being offered choices while being reminded of consequences for negative behavior.[23] This can be very rewarding to a child who is attempting new skills or is becoming more competent in self-care. The health care team can provide you with suggestions and recommendations when you are not sure what is appropriate for your child's health status.

Some parents become overprotective in an effort to prevent their child from being hurt. Protection requires a fine balance to ensure safety yet allow enough freedom for the child to grow and learn. Too much protection can hinder the developmental growth that promotes self-esteem, confidence, social skills and the chance to achieve goals. In addition continual restriction may aggravate the child's existing anger at his illness and treatments.[24]

ROBBY'S HOSPITAL CONTRACT

Date: _____

VITAL SIGNS	POINTS TO RECEIVE	POINTS EARNED
Robby will sit or lay quietly during vital signs in the morning and the evening.	1 Point each time vital signs are done.	_____
MORNING CARE		
Robby will bathe before 9:30 a.m. each morning when his mom sets up the wash basin at the bedside.	2 Points per day	_____
MEDICATIONS		
Robby will take his: Steroid (write in the name of the medication) at 8 a.m. Antibiotic at 3 & 9 a.m., and 3 & 9 p.m.	1 Point for each medication	_____
Total Points		_____
*Bonus Points		_____
Grand Total for the Day		_____

*Two bonus points can be earned each day, if all 8 points are earned for the full day.

—Robby can trade in 10 points for a single prize, or he may collect 140 points for a bonus prize.

Regular Prize	Bonus Prize
Baseball card pack of stickers a trip to the candy machine	radio head set new video game

Signed:
(Robby) _____   (Nurse) _____

(Mom) _____   (Doctor) _____

*This contract will be revised in two weeks so that Robby can make new choices for prizes.

Some parents tend to overindulge a child who is ill. Parents may feel the need to offer gifts and special treats to compensate for the child's suffering, as well as their own feelings of guilt over having to reinforce discipline. While occasional pampering can be used to raise morale, the frequency and manner in which overindulgence occurs can also overwhelm a child and frustrate his siblings. Overindulgence may be misinterpreted as giving up on a child's chances for recovery, or, if provided at the wrong times, may alter a child's perception of appropriate behavior. Children may take advantage of these opportunities to gain attention and gifts and to manipulate others. Overindulgence may focus too much attention on experiences that are easier to cope with if they are treated as something necessary and normal, such as ongoing daily treatments.[25] Maintaining a reward system without becoming overindulgent can be tricky, but your success can be gauged by your child's behavior.

For example, if your child expects a "treat" for complying with care, this can become frustrating (and costly) for you and can hamper your child's understanding of responsibility. His self-centeredness may increase and may be related to further difficulties at home. Spoiling or overindulging the ill child can also become an issue with friends, relatives, or teachers and should be discussed if concerns or frustrations develop. This is discussed in more detail in Chapter 8.

CONCERNS ABOUT RETURNING HOME

When your ill child is able to return home, you may feel reassured yet at the same time be frightened and apprehensive. Will your child's behavior return to normal? What changes have occurred that will require adjustment of existing schedules and family roles? What medical care will be required? What happens if your child gets ill again? Do you have enough expertise to provide care or determine when his health has changed and needs attention? What is expected of your child, and to what degree will life return to normal?

These are some of the many questions parents have when they return home with the ill child. It is reassuring to know, however, that "children and families have a better chance of achieving optimal psychosocial growth and development when the child is able to reside at home rather than in an institution" or hospital.[26]

When children return home from a hospitalization or clinic visit, some parents may notice additional changes in behavior. Some common reactions, particularly for younger children, include: nightmares, fear of strangers, fear of separation from a parent, temper tantrums, aggressive outbursts and attempting to avoid school.[27] Ongoing discussions about how your child feels and what he perceives is happening in his life may help to promote coping. Other suggestions for coping are provided throughout this book. Continued discussions with your child's physician or nurse will also provide more personal support and the opportunity to learn about local resources. Although additional changes in behavior can occur, your child will be less fearful and less distressed when the challenge of the hospital environment has been removed.

Home care can be beneficial for the family and child. However, the child's symptoms will not necessarily disappear when he comes home. New needs and responsibilities of the child and family members must be balanced with an attempt to reestablish previous routines when possible. Time must also be allotted for each person to have privacy as well as for fun times together. This allows everyone to recover emotionally and physically.

When medical care is required at home, you must determine a way to incorporate care into family routines. There are several suggestions for making treatment at home more tolerable. The first step is to familiarize yourself with the procedures. When learning to do treatments at home, remember that your child will be watching your reactions. If you appear uncomfortable or nervous, it may affect his willingness to participate in self-care.[28] Once you become comfortable you may find that treatments can become a valuable and special time for you and your child. (See table on page 111.)

When medical equipment is required in the home, it may seem very overwhelming and frightening at first, just as it had the first time it was encountered in the hospital. In the hospital, however, use of the equipment was supervised by hospital staff. When equipment is at home, who will be there to assure everything is working correctly? What happens in an emergency?

In addition to coordinating care services, one of the first steps is to learn how equipment works and who is available in emergencies. Health professionals, home care services or equipment companies should explain the equipment before your child's' discharge, and it is part of their job to make sure that you are comfortable with its use. Parents often become surprised at how easily they learn necessary information when the child has the opportunity to come home. Physicians, nurses, social workers, physical or respiratory therapists and health care service companies work together to provide your child with the necessary equipment and education to assure the safest and most comfortable transition to the home.

It is usually best to have information in written form to prevent misunderstanding of verbal instructions. Visits by certain professionals will usually be provided when first returning home. Periodic visits by differ-

SUGGESTIONS FOR MAKING TREATMENT AT HOME
MORE POSITIVE

Try to create a quiet and peaceful environment. Consider it a "special, quality time" just between you and your child (or other family members who may want to help).

If possible, develop a game to go with the treatment if it is not painful or stressful. One example for a young child would be a sing-along that labels parts of the body. This helps to teach the parts of the body and how the treatment is done.

To help your child feel more at ease, begin with a body massage. Softly stroke the arms, legs, or back and slowly work toward the area requiring treatment.

Have decorations or toys at eye level to occupy your child's attention during the treatment.

Even if a schedule is not required, perform the treatment at the same time(s) during the day or night to establish a routine for your child (such as after a nap or just before bed).

Establish an understanding about who will do what and when, allowing your child responsibility for some or all aspects of care when possible.

ent health care members will vary according to each child's case and should be scheduled before the child's discharge. Sometimes parents choose one person to act as coordinator of visits or equipment checks. It should be made clear who to contact when concerns arise regarding equipment, health care, insurance, or financial issues. The main thing parents should remember is that they are not alone.

In addition to maintaining the family, the coordination of care for the ill child can be frustrating if many people are involved and no coordinator is available to assist the parent. When discharge has been scheduled, there should be a conference with all health care team members and community service members who will be assisting the family. In addition, it may be helpful to have an insurance company representative or medical assistance representative present. When financial aid becomes necessary, social workers can look into medical eligibility and benefits from organizations such as the Crippled Children's Services. Financial aid policy varies from state to state.

To make sure the family will be able to care for the child at home and at the same time meet everyone else's needs, a social worker or nurse can help the parent to arrange a meeting to address the following questions: [29]

- What services will be needed and who will provide them?
- Who is responsible for referral for these services?
- Who will train the parent in medical treatments?
- Who will train the parent in the use of medical equipment?
- What equipment is needed?
- Who will provide health care visits?
- Who will provide equipment checks?
- What financial resources are available?
- When can another meeting be arranged to assure all needs are being met?
- Is there assistance with family needs such as transportation or child care?

By covering these topics and any other issues of concern to you or your family, you will feel less anxiety about what will happen when you arrive at home. If your child wants to participate in a meeting of this type he should do so. Your child's expectations could be clarified at this meeting. This can be especially important if he assumes that everything will return to normal when he gets home. The decision to allow your child to attend this type of meeting can be made by you, your child and the health care team. If a meeting is not suggested, you should request one, preferably a few days to a week before the child goes home.

Once your child does return home, family routines may need to be adjusted to accommodate educational needs, treatments and clinic visits. Parents may find it helpful to set daily schedules that include each family member's needs (similar to the schedule previously discussed), in addition to those of the child. Time should be allotted for family fun whenever possible to maintain morale and ongoing support for one another. Sometimes parents find it helpful to consult outside sources not directly involved with the child, such as family counselors or organizations specializing in the child's illness.

INSURANCE

Another area that has recently received attention is the difficulty parents encounter in getting or maintaining adequate insurance after their child has developed a life-threatening illness. This especially applies to illnesses or injuries that require ongoing medical care. Some parents who might wish to change jobs find that they must keep their current job to maintain their insurance coverage, because they would be unable to obtain new insurance that would cover "preexisting" conditions or illnesses. Some parents find that certain medical treatments, hospitalization, or doctor visits are not covered, sometimes after these services have already been provided. In some cases parents may assume that certain forms or referrals are automatically taken care of by health professionals, when in fact it is the parent's responsibility. Bills and statements accumulate and some parents begin to feel as if they are swimming in unforeseen debts.

The first step is to carefully examine health insurance policies to avoid surprises. This is usually not a priority when a child first becomes ill or injured, but early attention can help prevent many problems later. Phone calls to the insurance company and discussions with health care providers and social workers will help to explain terms and conditions to ensure proper coverage, or to outline what can be done if the family does not have adequate protection. Children with severe illnesses are usually not turned away from urgent medical care, and certain laws ensure this. Organizations related to the child's specific illness or injury can be especially helpful in directing the parent to resources that can help with financial and insurance problems. They can also provide information about state or federal laws that apply to the child's right to medical care and help the parent ensure that these rights are acknowledged.

Another source of information is your state or county health department. In some states, funds are available for the care of children with certain illnesses or disabilities, but eligibility for the funds varies. State government agencies or the local Veterans Administration may also provide information about federal laws or programs. One example is the Medical Assistance Program, which helps families with outstanding debts who need additional medical care. Thirty-four states now provide coverage for families that are considered "medically needy."[30] Other sources include private foundations or trust funds that have been established by people in the community to assist families with medical problems. Social workers, support groups or other organizations may provide a list of foundations in your area.

If you have insurance, it is important to organize a monthly file or system that will provide you with easy access to the following:[31]

- Statements (not bills, but a letter stating what medical care has been provided)
- Bills to be paid by the insurance company
- Bills to be paid by you (deductibles, balances or uncovered services)
- Information from the insurance company regarding changes in coverage

Review materials each month to make sure they have been properly handled by the hospital, physician, specialty services, and especially the insurance company. If you belong to a health maintenance organization, be sure that referrals or pre-authorizations are provided by the physician for each service. Keep a "medical diary" in which you note when referrals were made; this will serve as a documented source if the insurance company questions your referrals. There may not be a way to avoid financial pressures, but parents can prevent unanticipated bills or avoid mix-ups with insurance payments by keeping track of bills and statements. This information will also be very important for income tax deductions.

If you want to change your insurance, carefully review the new policy to make sure that ongoing medical care will be covered. Dr. Beryl Rosenstein, chairman of the Maryland Division of the Cystic Fibrosis Foundation, cautions parents about health maintenance organizations that strictly enforce where care is to be provided. He points out that clinics or programs that are designed to meet the special needs of certain illnesses or injuries may not be covered by this type of insurance, and thus the child may not have the opportunity to receive care that will maximize his recovery. Parents should be aware of these restrictions when pursuing any type of new insurance.

Parents cannot always avoid the problems of mounting bills or mix-ups between hospital and insurance payments, but they can make sure that bills are followed up and handled properly. Letting these problems "wait until later" only adds to the pressure on you, and unnecessary anxiety might distract you from devoting your full attention to your ill child and family. It is also important for parents to realize that people are available to help them, and legal and other problems can be avoided by consulting them.

SUPPORT GROUPS AND ORGANIZATIONS

Health professionals may not always be aware of your family's specific needs. At times, you must take the initiative to seek assistance from others. This assistance may sometimes be best provided by outside sources.

Some parents find it difficult to approach support groups or organizations because they want to be able to handle their child's care by themselves. They want to feel in control as well as be "an adequate parent" who does not need outside help. The child with a life-threatening illness has already been involved with so many people, and the parent may feel he has not had enough "hands-on" care of the child during hospitalization. He also may feel overburdened with the responsibility of care and have limited time and energy to leave the home.

When deciding whether or not to approach support groups or organizations, it may be helpful to understand some of the benefits they offer.[32]

BENEFITS OF SUPPORT GROUPS

THEY CAN INCREASE . . .	*THEY CAN PROVIDE . . .*	*THEY CAN PREVENT . . .*
Knowledge	Understanding	Feelings of isolation
Social interaction	Emotional support	Family difficulties
Feelings of usefulness	Resources for:	Misunderstandings
Hope	Education	Frustrations
	Child care	
	Transportation	
	Funds	
	Health professionals	

One misconception is that peer support groups are counseling or therapy groups. They are, in fact, groups of people with similar yet unique experiences who help educate and support each other. They are not involved in self-pity but instead provide strength for parents (or children) at a time when the many new issues of illness may make them feel overwhelmed. The groups can provide suggestions that health care professionals and extended family members may never have considered because they have not had to deal with the illness 24 hours a day, seven days a week.[33] They can also offer suggestions on how to deal with the professionals relating to specific illnesses or injuries. This kind of support can be invaluable in helping your family adapt to changes and prepare for the future. You in turn can gain satisfaction by offering the same help to others.

More formal organizations specializing in the child's illness offer parents other kinds of assistance. They have access to resources helpful to parents and can assist parents with career issues and finding specialized child care. They can also help parents understand financial issues such as tax deductions, financial aid and lobbying for new laws to assist families of ill children.

Support groups and organizations can also help in locating special camps, programs or peer groups for the ill child. These programs allow the child opportunities to learn and to simply have fun, they provide a healthy separation from parents and promote independence, and they foster personal growth through socialization and new friendships. They also may provide supplementary instruction for managing specific diseases or disabilities.

A list of resources provided in Appendix A will help you find an appropriate group to meet your own family's needs. Some organizations have local chapters in each state.

The more support your family has in helping your seriously ill child, the easier it will be to cope and adapt to the changes that are inevitable. The changes, while stressful, can be a positive, growing experience when discussed with others who understand what you are going through. It is up to you, however, to decide when and where to go for support based on your individual and family needs.

Notes

1. Dr. Raymond Mulherm, Director, Division of Psychology, St. Jude's Children's Hospital, Memphis Tennessee, Personal communication, May 1989.

2. S. E. Thorne and C. A. Robinson, "Health Care Relationships: The Chronic Illness Perspective," *Research in Nursing and Health* 11 (1988): 293–300.

3. W. R. McWhirter and J. P. Masel, *Pediatric Oncology: An Illustrated Introduction.* (Sydney: Williams & Wilkens and Associates, 1987), 116, 231.

4. M. N. Nathanson and G. Powers Monaco, "Meeting the Educational and Psychosocial Needs Produced by a Diagnosis of Pediatric/Adolescent Cancer," *Health Education Quarterly* 10 (1984): 1–112.

5. D. M. Orenstein, *Cystic Fibrosis: A Guide for Patient and Family*, (New York: Raven Press, 1989), 86–87.

6. J. M. Perrin and E. MacLean Jr., "Children With Chronic Illness: The Prevention and Dysfunction," *Pediatric Clinics of North America* 35 (December 1988): 1325–37.
   P. L. Rosenbaum, "Prevention of Psychosocial Problems in Children with Chronic Illness," *Canadian Medical Association Journal* 139(August 15, 1988): 293–95.
   S. Hewett, J. Newson, and E. Newson, *The Family and the Handicapped Child* (Chicago: Aldine Publishing Co., 1970), 76–113.
   A. Mattson and S. Gross, "Social and Behavioral Studies on Hemophiliac Children and Their Families," *Journal of Pediatrics* 68(1966): 952.

7. B. Sabbeth, "Understanding the Impact of Chronic Childhood Illness on Families," *Pediatric Clinics of North America* 31 (February 1984): 47–57.
   National Institutes of Health, *Coping with Cancer: A Resource for the Health Professional*, Publication no. 82-2080 (1982), 3–4, 47–53.

8. H. P. Greenwald, *Social Problems in Cancer Control* (Cambridge, Mass.: Ballinger Publishing Co., 1980), 15.

9. M. A. Chesler and O. A. Barbarin, *Childhood Cancer and the Family: Meeting the Challenge of Stress and Support* (New York: Brunner/Mazel, 1987), 223.

10. Rosenbaum, "Prevention of Psychological Problems in Children with Chronic Illness," 294.

11. M. N. Nathanson, "Meeting the Educational and Psychosocial Needs," p. 68; Association for the Care of Children's Health, *The Chronically Ill Child and Family in the Community* (1983): 2. S. K. Maul-Mellot and J. N. Adams, *Childhood Cancer: A Nursing Overview* (Boston: Jones and Bartlett Publishers, 1987).

12. Maul-Mellot and Adams, *Childhood Cancer*, p. 149–169.
A. T. McCollum, *Coping with Prolonged Health Impairment in Your Child* (Boston: Little Brown & Co., 1975), 22–23.
J. E. McElheny, "Parental Adaptation to a Child With Bronchopulmonary Dysplasia," *Journal of Pediatric Nursing* 4 (October 1989): 346–52.

13. A. E. Kazak, M. Reber, and L. Snitzer, "Childhood Chronic Disease and Family Functioning: A Study of Phenylketonuria," *Pediatrics* 81 (February 1988): 224–30.

14. National Institutes of Health, *Coping with Cancer*, 47–77.
Chesler and Barbarin, *Childhood Cancer and the Family.*
L. Pratt, *Family Structures and Effective Health Behaviors: The Energized Family* (Boston: Houghton Mifflin Co., 1976), 1–35.
Konrad and Ertle, *Pediatric Oncology*, p. 162–169.
Orenstein, *Cystic Fibrosis* p. 95–100.
J. Van Eys, ed., *The Truly Cured Child: The New Challenge in Pediatric Care* (Baltimore: University Park Press, 1976), 65–72.

15. Association for the Care of Children, *The Chronically Ill Child and Family in the Community*, (1983), 6.

16. Chesler and Barbarin, 141.

17. Ibid, 142.

18. Ibid, 144.

19. Dr. Raymond Mulherm, personal communication, May 1989.

20. Roberta Babbitt, Behavioral Analyst, Director of Out Patient Services, Kennedy Institute for Handicapped Children, Baltimore, Maryland, personal communication, April 1990.

21. S. B. Lansky and N. U. Cairns, "Psychiatric Syndromes in Pediatric Oncology Patients," *Psychiatric Medicine* 5(1987): 405–17.

22. Maul-Mellot and Adams, 160.

23. Dr. Linda Dahlquist, Ballor College of Medicine, personal communication, April 1990.

24. National Institutes of Health, *Coping with Cancer*, 67.

25. T. S. Langbaum and B. J. Rosenstein, *The Johns Hopkins Hospital Cystic Fibrosis Clinic Patient Handbook* (1985).

26. J. Kaufman and D. Hardy-Ribakow, "Home Care: A Model of a Comprehensive Approach for Technologically-Assisted Chronically Ill Children," *Journal of Pediatric Nursing* 2 (August 1987): 244.

27. Orenstein, 81–100.

28. E. K. Oremland, "Work Dynamics in Family Care of Hemophiliac Children," *Social Sciences & Medicine* 26(1988): 467–75.

29. N. Hobbs and J. M. Perrin, eds., *Issues in the Care of Children with Chronic Illness* (San Francisco: Jossey-Bass, 1985), 420–436.
    J. Kaufman and D. Hardy-Ribakow, "Home Care: A Model of a Comprehensive Approach for Technology-Assisted Chronically Ill Children," *Journal of Pediatric Nursing* 2(1987): 244–49.

30. R. E. K. Stein, ed., *Caring for Children with Chronic Illness: Issues and Strategies* (New York: Springer Publishing Company 1989).

31. R. Pincus, "Insurance Tips," *Candlelighters Quarterly Newsletter* 13 (Fall 1989): 5.
    Personal communication with families of cancer patients, August 1989.

32. Perrin and MacLean, "Children with Chronic Illness," 1333.
    Chesler and Barbarin, 189–191.

33. Chesler and Barbarin, 189.

7

SIBLINGS

UNDERSTANDING EFFECTS OF ILLNESS ON SIBLINGS

When a child with a serious illness has brothers or sisters, parents have additional concerns about how the siblings are affected: how they adjust, their changing emotions and changes in family routines. There are various views on the potential effects of serious illness on siblings. These effects can be governed by how each family functions, the family's experiences with health care professionals and the course of recovery. While opinions differ, there are consistent findings on the potential reactions of siblings and their capacity to understand illness. The following information may offer a basis for you to help your healthy children cope with serious illness or injury in a brother or sister.

HOW SIBLINGS MAY ADJUST

As siblings grow and learn together, it is evident that they can have a strong influence on one another. They may take turns acting as supporter, teacher, comforter and protector or conversely as instigator or rival. These roles and relationships can all be affected to different degrees when one of the children becomes seriously ill. In addition, siblings are faced with varying emotions and a disrupted home life that can also affect their school or social life. As discussed in Chapter 6, parents may go through stages in dealing with illness or injury of a child. It has also been suggested that siblings go through certain stages.[1]

At first, healthy siblings may have different degrees of awareness of how serious the illness actually is. The degree of awareness can be affected by their age, the amount of information offered, their parents' reactions, and the change in family routines. Siblings may only be aware that something is wrong, but may not understand that death is a possibility or even that death may take their brother or sister away. If they do realize the seriousness of the situation, they may become alarmed and react with feelings of shock or numbness. They may become increasingly sensitive to their parents' behavior in order to find out what is happening and whether or not they are being told everything.[2]

Once an ill child's condition has become stabilized, siblings may begin to feel that the child has a good chance for survival. The number of reminders of the illness, however, can affect how much the siblings will worry or think about the seriousness of the illness. Intermittent hospitalizations or clinic visits, sudden calls for the parents to rush to the hospital, or frequent treatments required at home can all serve to remind them of the possibility of death or that something can still go wrong. As these situations become less frequent, more siblings can become optimistic about the chances for survival and in turn may feel comfortable with resuming normal activities and plans.

COMMUNICATING WITH SIBLINGS

Open communication is essential for siblings to understand why their brother or sister is in the hospital. Just as parents want honesty from health professionals, brothers and sisters of ill children also need reassurance from parents about what is happening, why, and how it will affect them. The problem many parents encounter when talking with their healthy children is determining how much information should be offered in order to be reassuring yet not overwhelming. Just as with the ill child, parents feel it is their duty to protect their children from pain and suffering. As mentioned previously, children are surprisingly sensitive to their parents' behavior and body language, regardless of what is said. It has been found that parental anxiety can influence siblings' perceptions of the illness experience.[3] Siblings may receive conflicting signals from their parents, resulting in increased confusion and anxiety.[4] For example, parents may say the child is okay but are visiting the hospital more often. With a lack of information, siblings may begin to feel helpless and out of control, just as the ill child does. These feelings may lead to fear, jealousy and anger. The parent who avoids discussions about pain or other uncomfortable issues denies a real part of the ill child's life, and thus can make it more difficult for siblings to offer comforting support.

Discussions with siblings may be based on the same information offered to your ill child. You can respond to specific questions or base your conversation on information that will best help him prepare for any changes that may occur (such as when medical equipment is required at home).

For younger children (under the age of seven), less detailed information may minimize confusion and allow time for your child to absorb and comprehend what is being said. You should be available to answer questions, although you may need to initiate discussions with questions of your own, as siblings may not always express inner concerns unless they are directly asked.[5] They may be afraid of asking something that will upset their parent or may think that their worst fears will be confirmed. To open a discussion with your child, you can ask questions such as, "Do you know why your brother is sick?" or "Did you know I really miss you while I'm at the hospital?"

Older children may ask more detailed questions in an attempt to better understand what is happening and feel more in control of what they are able to do or say. If your teen is anxious about the ill child, you may be bombarded with questions (often at the most inopportune times). Adolescent siblings, however, may be particularly angered by any dishonesty or avoidance when parents attempt to protect them by withholding information. Adolescents want to be treated as adults. On the other hand, they may distance themselves from the situation and not ask questions at all. This may be their way of denying the illness, or they may be waiting for you to initiate the discussion.

A lack of communication between parents and siblings may have several possible effects, including reduced tolerance to changes, a sense of isolation, a lack of understanding of the illness and how it affects others and apprehension and stress. By avoiding discussion at times when siblings seek information, parents deny them the chance to express feelings and work through emotions or fears.

POSSIBLE REACTIONS OF SIBLINGS TO SERIOUS ILLNESS

FACTORS THAT MAY AFFECT BEHAVIOR

A sibling's reaction to a seriously ill brother or sister will vary with each illness or injury. As already discussed, the amount of information provided to a sibling has a significant effect on how he interprets different situations, and consequently how he will react.

If your ill child fluctuates between being very ill at times, yet is able to be at home and play at other times, it can create confusion and frustration for your healthy children. Explaining why this may happen (for example, infections might be harder for the ill sibling to fight, so he needs special medication in the hospital) can help to minimize the confusion. It might be difficult to overcome frustration, but allowing time with friends or visiting the hospital might help.

Opportunities for friends and school activities may become less frequent, however, due to problems arranging transportation or needing their help at home.

Another possible reason for behavior changes in siblings might be a lack of contact and interaction with the ill child, or on the other hand parents may force interaction before the siblings feel ready. Talking to, listening to, and watching your children together will help to determine if they need more or less involvement with your ill child.

◆ 123

POTENTIAL REACTIONS AND WAYS TO HELP

Because there are a number of factors that can affect how your children perceive the illness in a brother or sister, several types of behavior changes can result at any given time. While these changes can be normal responses to what your child is experiencing, they may occur in some siblings but may not in others. Individual coping strategies, in addition to individual perceptions of support and control, can also influence how your children will react.

Feelings and fears that siblings can experience are shown below:[6]

- Fear of catching the illness or becoming injured
- Guilt over how the child became ill or injured
- Fear of causing death or injury to the ill child
- Envy or jealousy of the attention the ill child receives
- Resentment of real or imagined responsibilities
- Being torn between own needs and loyalty to the family
- Fear of losing opportunities to do things
- Isolation from friends
- Anger toward parents, the ill child, or other family members
- Lack of control in family matters
- Isolation from the ill child
- Ongoing concern about potential survival of the ill child
- Embarrassment or shame over visible changes in the ill child's health

These feelings can be expressed through various changes in behavior similar to that of your ill child. Depending on his age, a healthy sibling may suddenly start having nightmares, having more temper tantrums, eating less and having trouble sleeping, and he may even begin to complain of symptoms similar to that of the ill brother or sister. A sibling may have increased discipline problems, may avoid friends, or may begin to have problems at school.[7]

For you to understand what your healthy children are feeling and thinking, you must make time to discuss their concerns. It has been found that when their questions go unanswered, siblings may create their own explanations based on their own experiences, the reactions of others (especially the parents) and fantasy thought.[8]

Open discussion throughout the course of the illness and treatments will help you to appreciate what your healthy children are feeling. It can be too overwhelming to cover too many issues at one time, so each discussion should be based on their current concerns.[9] Too much information can also raise anxiety about aspects of the illness the sibling may not have considered. It is important, however, that each child feel informed and prepared for any changes.

One research study found that parents and siblings did not always agree about the nature of the worries or concerns.[10] To clarify the sibling's concerns or understand changes in his life, discuss his own activities and school experiences to see how he has been affected. Discussing the reactions of your sibling's friends can also help him to cope with teasing or feeling isolated. It may help to explain that friends may not understand what has happened and what your family is going through, or that they may simply be afraid of saying the wrong thing. More information about friends is provided in Chapter 8.

Another way to learn how your healthy child is feeling is to use therapeutic play similar to that used with your ill child. Provide toys or play medical equipment for young siblings to explore. This stimulates them to ask any questions and communicate their fears, and lets them see in addition what their ill brother or sister is going through. Others can also provide this type of playtime when you or your partner can not be with them.

Sometimes younger siblings will be afraid that they will experience the illness or injury themselves. The best time to discuss this fear is during the early stages of your ill child's treatment, when you can dispel any misconceptions from the start. Another time these fears may be prominent is when the sibling becomes ill himself, such as getting the flu.[11] When a sibling becomes ill or injured, he may wonder why he does not receive as much attention, or why he receives no gifts. Reminding the sibling about the pain your ill child goes through to get better (or the things the ill child misses out on) might help to promote a better understanding about the difference in illnesses.

Preschool and young school-aged children may be afraid of "catching" what their brother or sister has and may fear that they too may die.[12] In addition, just as younger children who are ill may think that they have caused their illness by being "bad," siblings may similarly fear that they have caused their brother or sister to become ill. You can help prevent or discourage guilt that may arise as a result of these beliefs. You might say, for example, "Thank you for being so helpful while your sister is sick. Nobody did anything to cause it, but you mean a lot to him now that it has happened." You may need to discuss the topic of death with siblings in a similar manner to the ill child (if death is a concern for them).

Siblings who do not understand the illness may fear that they will harm or even kill the ill child when they are able to see and touch and play with him. Explaining what the ill child is able to do, how certain medical equipment helps maintain health, and what the sibling can do to help him may alleviate these fears. Family conferences can set the stage for everyone to discuss feelings when members are ready to talk openly. This is essential for siblings who are preoccupied with thoughts about death.

In some cases, healthy siblings react with envy or jealously when a parent needs to spend so much time with the ill child. These feelings occur in children of any age but vary in intensity. Younger children have stronger needs to be with their parents and are less able to understand the seriousness of an illness. They need more support in coping with separation from the parent and in understanding why it is necessary. Acknowledging that these feelings are normal (and are understood) may help them to feel less guilty. It can also be normal for a sibling to wish his brother or sister would die so that "things will go back to normal." He may not understand that if the ill child dies, he can not return. Death may viewed as a temporary solution or relief from current problems. While parents may even sometimes have these thoughts, it can be very difficult to talk about them. Siblings are comforted, however, when these feelings are acknowledged and understood by the parent.

Providing fun activities with favorite relatives or friends may help distract younger children from the absence of their parents, but ongoing discussions of their feelings will assure them that they are cared and thought about. Phone calls from or to the hospital can assure your child that he can still talk to you and that you are available. When you are able to spend time with siblings, set aside a mutually agreed upon "quality" time, to share activities such as going out for ice cream or playing a game. You can use that time, in a private, non-threatening environment, to discuss feelings, future plans and what is happening with the ill child. Siblings may also feel more comfortable about discussing their feelings with other brothers or sisters. You may learn more about their feelings from private discussions with each child, but you should not force siblings to break confidence among one another unless you feel it is essential to their well-being.

As a result of changes in your family routines, siblings may begin to resent having to do more around the house and getting less support for what they want to do, or the fact that you are no longer doing what you used to do. It is important that you acknowledge what they are doing to help, even if it is done differently or is not done as well as expected. Praise can increase their desire to help.

Siblings may also begin to feel torn between their family responsibilities and their own plans and activities. Younger children, who are so eager to explore and learn new things, may now feel confined or restricted. They thrive on praise from parents and like to feel helpful but are also so eager to play. When they become confused or distressed by having these conflicting feelings, they may begin to fluctuate between being "good" and being defiant. Older children have the strong need to socialize with friends but still feel loyalty to the family. They, too, may have conflicts over how to spend their time and meet their responsibilities. Open discussions will help to air their grievances, acknowledge their needs and establish expectations for responsibility.

Siblings may become concerned about lost opportunities, such as family vacations put on hold, missing outside activities or having less time for school projects. This can be especially troublesome for school-aged children and adolescents who value being with their friends and are more concerned about being left out. They also lose the opportunity to be "like" their friends at a time when they need to feel a part of a group outside of the family. Whenever possible, changes to siblings' routines should be minimized but it is important to emphasize that their plans should remain flexible.

As previously mentioned, siblings may feel they are being left out of experiences with the ill brother or sister. When a brother or sister is hospitalized, siblings may enjoy phoning the hospital room, making get well cards, giving a present, writing a letter, writing a story for the brother or sister or even making a tape-recorded message to be played in the hospital. These provide alternative ways to communicate if the sibling is afraid to interact directly with the ill child or if hospital rules do not allow visits by young children.

Some siblings become angry as a result of changes that are unavoidable and inevitable. In some cases anger is directed toward the ill child for getting sick. You may become the focus of anger when you need to spend so much time away from home or must catch up on household tasks when you are at home. You may also bear the brunt of angry outbursts when siblings become angry about things that are happening at school or with friends. This behavior is easier to accept and tolerate if you remember not to take it personally. Patience is important, yet discipline should still be enforced when it is needed (as with the ill child) to make sure that the siblings understand what is expected, what behavior is appropriate and how to redirect their anger. Providing outlets to express the anger as suggested in chapters 4 and 6 can also apply to siblings. Acknowledging that these feelings can be normal and healthy will give the siblings the message that they are not "terrible" people.

Siblings may feel they lack control in family matters. When chores or family tasks are decided, siblings should be allowed to take part in the decision-making process so that they can voice any plans they may have and discuss whether or not they feel overwhelmed or whether someone has not been doing his share of household chores. They may also feel overlooked when they are not told about treatment plans for the ill child or what will happen when the ill child comes home. It may also help to prepare them in advance for sudden changes, such as an unexpected hospitalization or doctor's visit.

Siblings often worry about their brother or sister during treatment and when the child comes home from the hospital. Just as parents worry about the ill child even after recovery, siblings have ongoing concerns. One study has found that school-aged children have stated that the most difficult part of having an ill sibling is worrying about them.[13] The worry is expressed in any number of ways, including complaining of similar symptoms, distancing themselves from the ill child, having nightmares or crying frequently. Acknowledging their concern and providing ongoing information can help them to work through these feelings.

In some cases, especially when the ill child returns home or to school, siblings will feel ashamed of or embarrassed by changes in him that are noticeable to others. Even though they are happy that their sibling is recovering, mental or physical changes may be difficult for them to discuss with friends. They may not invite friends to visit as frequently, they may avoid the sibling in public or at school or they may find themselves in fights to defend the sibling. It may help to discuss potential reactions of others and how to handle these situations before they occur. More suggestions are provided in Chapter 8.

SUMMARY OF SUGGESTIONS FOR HELPING SIBLINGS

On page 129 is a list of suggestions for helping siblings with an ill brother or sister. Discussions with the health care team, family members, the ill child, and of course with each sibling will help to determine what is best for your own family. No one can determine exactly how each person will be affected, and only time and trial and error will decide what will help everyone concerned.[14]

POSITIVE EFFECTS OF AN ILL BROTHER OR SISTER ON SIBLINGS

While much research has focused on the negative effects of serious illness on healthy siblings, positive outcomes have been noted as well.

Arrange for siblings to visit the hospital or accompany the ill child to doctor or clinic visits.

Be firm with relatives and friends about spoiling the ill child with gifts and attention.

Provide time for each sibling and for family time together.

If children like to help out at home, allow them to choose tasks and acknowledge their efforts.

When friends or relatives offer to help out, be sure your children are comfortable with them. Explain how long they will be there and where you will be.

Provide updated information about the ill child's condition, expected homecoming, and what changes may occur.

Provide opportunities for "medical" or therapeutic play.

Acknowledge their feelings and assure them that they are normal, perhaps explaining that you have felt the same way.

Acknowledge strengths and achievements of each sibling.

Consider differences between siblings and remember that each will set his own pace for learning and becoming involved.

Discuss what is happening in their own lives.

Discuss concerns about behavior changes or school problems with the medical staff and the sibling's own doctor.

Avoid changing discipline methods for the sibling or ill child.

Avoid setting high expectations for healthy siblings.

Avoid using comparative words such as "better" or "worse," when discussing the ill child's condition. For example, "Your brother will be using a wheelchair now because his legs work *differently* than before and he needs more help to move around."

Recent research has sought to understand how siblings and families successfully cope in order to help others learn the best way to handle the stress and frustration encountered during diagnosis, treatment and recovery.

Positive effects on siblings have been found to include more tolerance, compassion and a better understanding of prejudice.[15] When a brother or sister becomes ill, siblings learn how priorities may change and how needs are met in different ways. They learn that there may be reasons why people act differently, and they may become more tolerant when things are not going their way or when someone is not as nice.

Siblings also may begin to take pride in helping their parents. It can be especially rewarding for them to take part in caring for the ill brother or sister once they have become comfortable with the illness and treatment.[16] As long as they are not overwhelmed with too many tasks, siblings learn about responsibility and gain a feeling of independence.

When a sibling has adapted and accepted the illness, he may become a more sensitive and caring person, lasting into adulthood.[17] He may be less apt to criticize others and be more sensitive to their needs.

Notes

1. K. M. Brett and E. M. B. Davies, "What Does It Mean: Sibling and Parental Appraisals of Childhood Leukemia," *Cancer Nursing* 11(1988): 329–38.

2. Ibid, 336.

3. Ibid., 335.
   M. Seligman, "Siblings of Handicapped Persons," in M. Seligman, ed., *The Family with a Handicapped Child: Understanding and Treatment* (New York: Grune & Stratton, 1983), 147–174.

4. L. Pearlman and K. Scott, *Raising the Handicapped Child* (Englewood Cliffs, N.J.: Prentice Hall, 1981).

5. Brett and Davies, 335–336.

6. P. Isles, "Children and Cancer: Healthy Siblings' Perceptions During the Illness Experience," *Cancer Nursing* 2(1979): 371–77.
   B. Sabbeth, "Understanding the Impact of Chronic Illness on Families," *Pediatric Clinics of North America* 31 (February 1984): 47–57.
   Seligman, "Siblings of Handicapped Persons, 289–90.
   C. L. Walker, "Stress of Coping in Siblings of Childhood Cancer Patients," *Nursing Research* 37(July/August 1988): 208–12.

7. Association for the Care of Children's Health, "The Chronically Ill Child and Family in the Community," (1983), 7.

8. Brett and Davies, 336.

9. Carr-Gregg and White, "Siblings of Pediatric Cancer Patients," pp. 62–68.

10. E. M. Menke, "The Impact of a Child's Chronic Illness on School-aged Siblings," *Children's Health Care* 15(Winter 1987): 132–40.

11. Seligman, 289.

12. C. Pochedly, ed., *Cancer Therapy in Children* (Thorofare, N.J.: Slack, 1983).

13. Menke, "The Impact of a Child's Chronic Illness," 135.

14. Carr-Gregg and White, 63–66.

K. K. Scheiber, "Developmentally Delayed Children: Effects on the Normal Sibling," *Pediatric Nursing* 15(Jan./Feb. 1989): 42–44.

Personal communication with Dr. Raymond Mulherm, Director of the Division of Psychology; St. Jude's Children's Hospital, Memphis, Tennessee, May 1989.

15. F. K. Grossman, *Brothers and Sisters of Retarded Children* (Syracuse: Syracuse University Press, 1972), 176.

16. Seligman, 290.

17. N. Hobbs, J. M. Perrin, and H. T. Ireys, eds., *Chronically Ill Children and Their Families* (San Francisco: Jossey-Bass, 1985), 94–95.

8

FRIENDS AND FAMILY

TELLING OTHERS ABOUT THE ILLNESS

SHOULD YOU BURDEN OTHERS WITH YOUR PROBLEMS?

Among their many personal and family challenges, parents begin to realize that others in their lives are also affected when their child has a serious illness or injury. Relatives, close friends, neighborhood friends, church or synagogue members, school personnel, coworkers and people in the community will eventually learn about the change in the child's health. Each person's response will vary—from acceptance to denial—depending on previous experiences and perception of the prognosis. People talk, and whether or not they hear it from you, others will learn about the illness or injury.

You may wish to tell certain people but be afraid of burdening them with your problems. If you tell everyone, you may be afraid they will think you are looking for sympathy. If you only tell some and not others, will feelings get hurt? What will the people you have told say to your children? Will they offer support?

You may get a lot of support from family and friends, but informing them of the illness as well as your needs can be stressful. Your relationship with each person will determine how much you tell them, whether you say anything at all or whether you "get everything off your chest." You will probably try to guess how they will react before saying anything. When you do discuss it, you may find some people will "stereotype" the illness; they do not realize that each child with a serious illness can have a different recovery course and that your own child's personality and experiences can influence the way he will adapt. Some people will react calmly, while others will be more emotional. You may be unsure of how someone will react and be unable to decide what to say.

WHY SOME FAMILIES SHARE THEIR EXPERIENCES WITH OTHERS

People will have different reactions to illness, as well as expectations for recovery, based on their own experience. Parents and children can help prevent false expectations or fears by providing factual information about the illness or injury to others. In doing so, parents and their children can help establish more secure relationships of support and understanding. For families who openly discuss what is happening in their lives it often becomes easier to ask for support, or others offer support more openly and more in line with what the family needs.

In order not to incur sympathy, some families treat the illness or injury as a "fact of life," and one that does not affect *all* of their goals and activities.

INVOLVEMENT OF FAMILY MEMBERS

Parents sometimes have conflicting emotions about how family members should be involved, how much they can help, and how much they should leave to the parents. Relatives can offer emotional support at a time when parents feel confused and overwhelmed. Grandparents, aunts and uncles or other close family members can also be a significant support for siblings who need attention at a time when parents are focused on the ill child. By caring for the siblings or the home, they can give the parents some time to restore themselves emotionally and physically.

Family members can also offer suggestions that parents may not think of when concentrating on other matters. For example, an aunt may provide a new activity to entertain siblings while the mother is at the hospital. Relatives also may take over some of the mundane tasks such as household chores or transportation. Some relatives may even be able to provide help with temporary financial assistance, making certain each party understands the terms of the aid.

By concentrating on the many ways relatives can help, you may be less apt to see their involvement as "interference." Sometimes you may feel that family members interfere with inappropriate suggestions or take over tasks that you actually want or need to do. It is important to make everyone aware of your needs. Family members may simply be expressing their need to feel involved by offering their "idea" of support.

Dealing with their concerns may be frustrating at first. Relatives may ask questions over and over again, or they may even call a nurse or doctor directly in an attempt to understand and accept the illness or injury. Providing pamphlets, or making friends available to explain more details, can lessen the strain on you.

It can also be frustrating when family members attempt to help but do not fully understand your wishes or suggestions. They may unintentionally do more harm than good. You may begin to feel that your privacy has been invaded, or that family members are overindulging your ill child, which in turn can create additional problems for you. Informal "contracts" can be established by simply writing down your wishes as well as your reasons for them. For example, you may find it beneficial to talk about the need for continued discipline, or warn that overindulging your ill child can hurt the siblings' feelings. Emphasize that spending time with the ill child (but even more so with siblings) is more beneficial than any material rewards, which would only temporarily provide happiness.[1]

Occasionally, family members may be critical of you. This can be especially upsetting during stressful times when you are simply trying to cope with the illness or injury. Criticizing or blaming may be one way in which family members try to justify why the child has been ill or injured. Just as you may have felt the need to rationalize what has happened, but have since accepted it, your relatives may just be beginning to work through similar feelings.

They may also disagree with treatment plans. They may be responding to their emotions rather than an understanding of the facts. They may also associate the situation with a previous experience, or something they have heard about the illness or injury. In trying to prevent problems, they may unintentionally create them. They usually are not aware that they are "criticizing."

Calm, tactful and open communication may help them to realize their behavior. If it seems that they are intentionally being critical, simply tell them that their comments are not helpful but are upsetting and that you prefer to end the discussion. It may help to relay these problems to other family members who can work out negative feelings with those who are being difficult and leave you to the tasks at hand. When appropriate, it may also be very beneficial to have a family conference with the medical staff, who can cover aspects of diagnosis, treatments and the recovery process.

On the other hand, it may seem that family members are uncaring or more distant than usual. This can be hard to understand because family is usually expected to be supportive. They may not want to interfere and prefer to wait for you to initiate contact or they may be afraid of saying the wrong thing and triggering negative feelings by talking about something that will relate to the ill child.

They may also have misconceptions about the illness (for example, that it is incurable) and fear certain death. Older relatives who face the reality of death may have a more difficult time accepting the illness, and thus might not talk about it. Others may be denying the seriousness of the illness to protect themselves or you by not talking. Some relatives may feel numb (or unsure of what they are feeling) and may need time to work through their own feelings.

For many of the same reasons already stated regarding communication between children and partners, family members will only be able to understand aspects of the illness that have been discussed with them. This can be difficult when you must convey information over and over again at a time when all you want to do is focus on getting things back to normal. You must decide what they need to know and leave out details that will create anxiety or more confusion.

You must remember, however, that only you can realize the extent of the changes that have occurred in your own family life. Others will react based on their own perceptions or what they have been told. It is up to you to explain how you feel and what you need from relationships with others.[2]

INVOLVEMENT OF FRIENDS AND CO-WORKERS

During this time, parents may find that relationships with close friends and co-workers are strained. Parents may feel that these friendships are being "tested," or that only "true" friends are staying in touch.

It may be up to you to establish contact with some friends for several reasons. Some friends will feel it is a time for family and will assume that you will call when you are up to conversations with others. Just like some relatives, friends may be unsure of what to say or will be afraid of prying into personal business. Staying away may actually be an attempt to show consideration for your privacy; they may not realize that they can be more supportive by contacting you. You can establish guidelines by initiating contact with phone calls or letters, mentioning when you would like to see or hear from others. At times when you need your privacy simply tell them "We have family time every night after 8:00 P.M.; we appreciate phone calls before that time."

If you feel comfortable with others knowing about the illness or injury but are tired of talking about it, you may ask those who you have told to "pass along" the information. If you feel like talking, or simply want to be treated normally again, think of a way to initiate conversations. One parent who returned to work after her daughter had been hospitalized for leukemia decided to "break the ice" with co-workers by placing a sign on her desk that said, "I smile too."

At times, parents may prefer contact with a close friend to some relatives. In times of stress, certain personalities appear to deal with the situation better than others. In addition, you may be concerned about burdening certain relatives who may be having their own difficulties, or perhaps the siblings are closer to a family friend than a relative.

If this is the case for you, and you are afraid of hurting someone's feelings, you must decide what is best for your family and put their needs first. While some may feel hurt, explaining why certain people are more involved than others will help to ease tensions and resentment. Emphasize that others should respect your wishes, as you are doing the best you can to support your family. For those who offer to help, think of things they can do, such as calling organizations for information, buying groceries, or calling other family members to let them know what is happening. If they become too intrusive, let them know you appreciate their concern and all they have done, but now you need some time alone with your family. Parents can maintain close and supportive relationships with family members when they are caring yet assertive.

DEALING WITH THE CHILD'S OR SIBLINGS' FRIENDS

The ill child and his siblings may have similar experiences with their own friends. There are, however, several differences in how children deal with their peers.

Depending on their developmental level, providing factual information to friends and school teachers can benefit children in several ways. As discussed in Chapter 4, children can help foster understanding by informing their teachers, who in turn can help educate classmates. Informing others can help minimize fear and misconceptions (and thus minimize teasing).

It is up to each family, however, to determine how much information they wish to share, as well as how many people really need to know. If appropriate, you should emphasize that your child is not to be labeled (such as "Johnny is the cancer kid"). It is important to convey that your child's life needs to be normalized, and what should be expected of him and his siblings. If you have been able to obtain pamphlets or brochures share them with close friends and schoolmates who may be reassured by reading about the illness. To prevent your children from having to explain things over and over again, they may let friends pass information on to others, emphasizing that they are open to questions.

When parents encourage experiences outside of the home (such as going to school or joining in community activities), their ill child and siblings may feel awkward or anxious at first. The children can overcome this initial discomfort, however, and benefit from increased self-esteem, heightened productivity, and a better sense of what they can do.[3] They can feel part of a group again (important for emotional and social development) and begin a healthy separation from parents and family after a period of confinement. A non-threatening way to begin contact early in the illness or the recovery period, is to make phone calls or write letters, which maintain contact at a safe distance.

Children's desires to share information about themselves vary from child to child and can change over time. Outgoing young children may take pride in providing details about an illness and injury, showing off new words and new medical care skills. Older children may fear being different from friends and may wish to be more secretive about the illness.[4] Parents can discuss each child's feelings, acknowledging that each may have different fears or ways of coping. Each child may also have different expectations of a friend's reactions, based on previous interactions or past experiences.

Some diseases or injuries carry a certain stigma that may be based on misconceptions or inaccurate information. For example AIDS, or acquired immune deficiency syndrome, is frightening to people who do not understand how it is transmitted. Children with hemophilia or other conditions who were given blood transfusions before screening began in 1985 may have acquired AIDS as a result of their medical care, yet they are still stereotyped and teased about having AIDS. The ill child and his siblings may hesitate to discuss such an illness with friends, fearing that they will be discriminated against by their friends, neighbors and community.

People may also have fears of other illnesses or injuries. Young children may be afraid they will catch an illness such as cancer, cystic fibrosis or kidney disease. Some might believe that all brain injuries result in paralysis or "brain death." Educating friends is essential to successfully mainstream your children back into the community. Preparing your family to discuss the illness or injury will help them be more comfortable in approaching those they wish to tell.

It helps to keep the tone of any discussion on a straightforward, factual level. Accentuate positive aspects, such as what the child is able to do. Explain any changes in the child's appearance or functioning, for example if speech is slow or slurred, sometimes others may interpret this as a form of brain damage that affects comprehending what is said, when in fact the child hears and understands, but only has difficulty talking back. Emphasize how others can talk to or help the child on a level appropriate for him. Listen to and observe your children to see if they are open to questions from others. The child should not be forced to talk about the illness if not ready, or if too many people are asking questions. Emphasize, however, that if the illness is treated more as a secret, there is a greater chance for others to be fearful. It also denies a part of the child's life that he may need to talk about in order to accept it his or herself.

To help your children cope with fears about relating to others, begin by talking to them about their day with friends. It may take time for some children to openly talk about their experiences, and others may wish to handle everything by themselves. You know each child's personality and can sense if something is bothering one of them. Playing with your children provides opportunities to talk in a less threatening manner, as well as providing time to offer suggestions without "lecturing."

Talking to teachers and friends' parents about your children can also be enlightening but must be done in such a way that your children will not feel you are interfering or "mothering" too much. In order to maintain their trust, you must not appear to be going behind their back.

By providing time and preparation to guide your children, you can allow them to return to normal activities at their own pace and on their own terms. All children go through growing pains in order to develop their self-image. Although it is frustrating and at times upsetting, conquering their fears and overcoming difficult relationships with the support of their parents can build their confidence and understanding.

Notes

1. National Institutes of Health, *Taking Time: Support for People With Cancer and the People Who Care About Them*, Publication no. 87-2761 (April 1987).

2. M. A. Chesler and O. A. Barbarin, *Childhood Cancer and The Family: Meeting the Challenge of Stress and Support* (New York: Brunner/Mazel, Inc., 1987), 194–208.

3. I. D. Bullard and J. T. Dohnal, "The Community Deals With the Child Who Has a Handicap," *Nursing Clinics of North America* 19(June 1984):309–18.

4. E. K. Oremland, "Work Dynamics in Family Care of Hemophilic Children," *Social Science & Medicine* 26(1988): 467–75.

APPENDIX

RESOURCES

Adolescent Autonomy Project
Children's Rehabilitation Center
2270 Ivy Road
Charlottesville, VA 22901

Adolescent Employment Readiness Center (for adolescents 12–19)
Children's Hospital National Medical Center
111 Michigan Avenue N.W.
Washington, DC 20010
202-745-3203

The American Association of Marriage and Family Counselors
225 Yale Avenue
Claremont, CA 91711

American Cancer Society
777 Third Avenue
New York, NY 10017
212-371-2900

American Diabetes Association
1660 Duke Street
Alexandria, VA 22314

American Heart Association
7320 Greenville Avenue
Dallas, TX 75231

American Kidney Fund
6110 Executive Boulevard
Suite 1010
Rockville, MD 20852
1-800-638-8299

American Lung Association
1740 Broadway
New York, NY 10019

American Medical Association
535 N. Dearborn Street
Chicago, IL 60610

American Psychiatric Association
1200 17th Street N.W.
Washington, DC 20036

Arizona Consortium for Children with Chronic Illness
P.O. Box 2128
Phoenix, AZ 85001

Arthritis Foundation
3400 Peachtree Road N.E.
Atlanta, GA 30326

Association for the Care of Children's Health
Organizing Support Groups for Parents of Children with Chronic Illness
and Handicapping Conditions, Parent Resource Directory:
3615 Wisconsin Avenue N.W.
Washington, DC 20016

Association for Persons with Severe Handicaps
Liz Lindley, Executive Director
7010 Roosevelt Way N.E.
Seattle, WA 98115
206-523-8446

Camps for Children with Special Needs and Their Families
Parents' Guide to Accredited Camps
American Camping Association
100 Bradford Woods
Martinsville, IN 46151

Camp Kaleidoscope (for children with chronic illnesses)
P.O. Box 2916
Duke University Medical Center
Durham, NC 27710

Camp Needlepoint
Contact the American Diabetes Association
3005 Ottawa Avenue South
St. Louis Park, MN 55416

Camp Ozawizeniba (for children and youth with epilepsy)
2701 University Avenue S.E.
Suite 106
Minneapolis, MN 55406

Camp Superkids
1829 Portland Avenue
Minneapolis, MN 55404

Cancer Care, Inc.
1180 Avenue of the Americas
New York, NY 10036
212-302-2400

Cancer Hopefuls United for Mutual Support
3310 Rochambeau Avenue
Bronx, NY 10467
212-655-7566

Cancer Information Services
1-800-422-6237

Candlelighters Foundations (for children with cancer)
Grace Powers Monaco, National Liaison Chairperson
1312 18th Street N.W.
2nd Floor
Washington, DC 20003
202-483-9100

Child and Family Support Project
Children's Hospital Medical Center
4800 Sand Point Way
Seattle, WA 98105

Children's Defense Fund
122 C Street N.W.
Suite 400
Washington, DC 20001
202-628-8787

Children in Hospitals
31 Wilshire Park
Needham, MA 02192

Children's Liver Foundation
76 South Orange Avenue
South Orange, NJ 07079
201-761-1111

Chronic Illness Teaching Program
Department of Pediatrics and Human Development
B-240, Life Sciences Building
Michigan State University
East Lansing, MI 48824

Clearinghouse on the Handicapped
Office of Special Education and Rehabilitative Services
Department of Education
Room 3106 Switzer Building
230 C Street S.W.
Washington, DC 20202

Compassionate Friends (for patients with cancer)
P.O. Box 1347
Oakbrook, IL 60521

Coordination of Care for Chronically Ill Children Program
New York State Department of Health
Tower Building, Room 878
Empire State Plaza
Albany, NY 12237

Cystic Fibrosis Foundation
National Office
6931 Arlington Road
Bethesda, MD 20814
1-800-FIGHT CF

Digestive Diseases
Box NDOIC
Bethesda, MD 20892
202-296-1138

Division of Maternal and Child Health
U.S. Public Health Service
5600 Fishers Lane
Rockville, MD 20857

Epilepsy Foundation of America
4351 Garden City Drive
Landover, MD 20785

Federation for Children with Special Needs
312 Stuart Street, 2nd Floor
Boston, MA 02116

Grief Institute
P.O. Box 623
Englewood, CO 80151

Helping Grandparent Program
King County ARC
2230 Eighth Avenue
Seattle, WA 98121

Home-Based Support Services for Chronically Ill Children
    and Their Families
Tower Building, Room 878
Empire State Plaza
Albany, NY 12237

Hydrocephalus Dystrophy Association
810 Seventh Avenue
New York, NY 10019
212-586-0808

Infant and Child Special Care, Inc.
402 Wall Street
Valparaiso, IN 46304

International Diabetes Center
Park Nicollet Medical Foundation
5000 West 39th Street
Minneapolis, MN 55416

Juvenile Diabetes Foundation
23 East 26th Street
New York, NY 10010

Leukemia Society of America, Inc.
Meade P. Brown, Executive Director
211 East 43rd Street
New York, NY 10017
212-573-8484

Make Today Count (for patients with cancer)
P.O. Box 222
Osage Beach, MI 65065
314-348-1619

Mothers of Asthmatics, Inc.
10875 Main Street
Suite 210
Fairfax, VA 22030

Muscular Dystrophy Association
Robert Ross, Executive Director
810 Seventh Avenue
New York, NY 10019
212-586-0808

National Amputation, Inc.
12–45 150th Street
Whitestone, NY 11357
718-767-0596

National Association for Sickle-Cell Disease, Inc.
3460 Wilshire Boulevard
Suite 1012
Los Angeles, CA 90010

National Association of Social Workers
1425 H Street N.W., Suite 600
Washington, DC 20005

National Cancer Foundation, Inc.
Irene Buckley, Executive Director
One Park Avenue
New York, NY 10016
212-679-5700

The National Easter Seal Society for Crippled Children and Adults
2023 W. Ogden Avenue
Chicago, IL 60612

National Foundation for Childhood Arthritis
2424 Pennsylvania Avenue N.W.
Washington, DC 20037

National Head Injury Foundation
18A Vernon Street
Framingham, MA 01701

National Heart and Lung Institute
Bethesda, MD 20014

National Hemophilia Foundation
19 W. 34th Street
New York, NY 10001

National Information Center for Children and Youth with Handicaps
P.O. Box 1492
Washington, DC 20013
703-893-6061

National Information Center for Handicapped Children and Youth
Delores John, Director
P.O. Box 1492
Washington, DC 20013
703-522-3332

National Institute of Mental Health
5600 Fishers Lane
Rockville, MD 20852

National Kidney Foundation
2 Park Avenue
New York, NY 10016

National Multiple Sclerosis Society
208 E. 42nd Street
New York, NY 10017

National Organization for Rare Diseases
P.O. Box 8923
New Fairfield, CT 06812
203-746-6518

National Reye's Syndrome Foundation
426 N. Lewis
Bryan, OH 43506
419-636-2679

National Spinal Cord Injury HOTLINE
2201 Argonne Drive
Baltimore, MD 21218
1-800-526-3456

Office of Cancer Communications
National Cancer Institute
Building 31, Room 10A18
Bethesda, MD 20205

Office of Special Education and Rehabilitation Services
U.S. Department of Education
330 E Street S.W.
Switzer Building
Washington, DC 20202
202-732-1273

Osteogenesis Imperfecta Foundation, Inc.
P.O. Box 838
Manchester, NH 03105

Parents of Premature and High Risk Infants International, Inc.
c/o C.A.S.E.
33 W. 42nd Street
New York, NY 10036

Parents of Premies
9307 Doris Drive
Ft. Washington, MD 20744

PATHFINDER
(Improving systems of care for medically vulnerable children)
5000 W. 39th Street
Minneapolis, MN 55416

Pediatric Projects Incorporated
P.O. Box 1880
Santa Monica, CA 90406
213-828-8963
714-496-4134

Pediatrics for Parents (monthly newsletter on general health issues)
Box 1069
Bangor, ME 04401

Ronald McDonald Houses-Coordinator
(for housing accommodations near hospitals)
c/o Golin/Harris Communications, Inc.
500 N. Michigan Avenue
Chicago, IL 60611
312-836-7129

Sick Kids Need Involved People (SKIP) [for Technology Dependent
Children]
216 Newport Drive
Severna Park, MD 21146
301-647-0164

Special Needs Parent Information Network
P.O. Box 2067
Augusta, ME 04330
1-800-325-0220

Spina Bifida Association of America
343 S. Dearborn Street
Suite 319
Chicago, IL 60604

Spinal Cord Injury Association
600 W. Cummings Parkway
Suite 2000
Woburn, MA 01801
1-800-962-9629

United Cancer Council, Inc.
Suite 340
650 East Carmel Drive
Carmel, IN 46032
317-844-6627

United Cerebral Palsy Association, Inc.
330 W. 34th Street
New York, NY 10001

Very Special Arts (creative learning for children with special needs)
Education Office
John F. Kennedy Center for the Performing Arts
Washington, DC 20566
202-662-8899

BIBLIOGRAPHY

Ack, M. "Psychosocial Effects of Illness, Hospitalization, and Surgery." *Journal of the Association for the Care of Children's Health* 11(Spring 1983): 132–36.

Adams, D. W., and Deveau, E. J. *Coping with Childhood Cancer: Where Do We Go From Here?* Reston, Va.: Reston Publishing Company, 1984.

American Cancer Society. *When Your Brother or Sister Has Cancer.* 1984.

American Cancer Society. *Parents' Handbook on Leukemia.* 1987.

Association for the Care of Children's Health. *The Chronically Ill Child and Family in the Community.* Washington, D.C., 1983.

Association for the Care of Children's Health. *Caring for Your Hospitalized Baby.* Washington, D.C., 1984.

Association for the Care of Children's Health. *Preparing Your Child for Repeated or Extended Hospitalizations.* 3rd printing. 1987.

Baum, B. J., and Baum, E. S. "Psychosocial Challenges of Childhood Cancer." *Journal of Psychosocial Oncology* 7(1989): 119–29.

Betz, C. L., and Poster, E. C. "Children's Concepts of Death: Implications for Pediatric Practice." *Nursing Clinics of North America* 19(June 1984):341–49.

Brett, K. M., and Davies, E. M. B. "What Does It Mean?: Sibling and Parental Appraisals of Childhood Leukemia." *Cancer Nursing* 11(1989): 329–38.

Broome, M. E. "The Relationship Between Children's Fears and Behavior During a Painful Event." *Journal of the Association for the Care of Children's Health* 14(Winter 1986):142–45.

Bullard, I. D., and Dohnal, J. T. "The Community Deals With the Child Who Has A Handicap." *Nursing Clinics of North America* 19(June 1984): 309–18.

Carr-Gregg, M. and White, L. "Siblings of Pediatric Cancer Patients: A Population at Risk." *Medical & Pediatric Oncology* 15(1987):62–68.

Caty, S.; Ritchie, J. A.; and Ellerton, M. L. "Mothers' Perceptions of Coping Behaviors in Hospitalized Preschool Children." *Journal of Pediatric Nursing* 4(December 1989):403–10.

Chesler, M. A., and Barbarin, O. A. *Childhood Cancer and the Family: Meeting the Challenge of Stress and Support*. New York: Brunner/Mazel, 1987.

Chekryn, J.; Deegan, M.; and Reid, J. "Impact on Teachers When A Child with Cancer Returns to School." *Journal of the Association for the Care of Children's Health* 15(Winter 1987):161–65.

Conaster, C. "Preparing the Family for Their Role During Treatment." *Cancer* 58(1986):508–11.

Copeland, D. R.; Pfefferbaum, B.; and Stovall, A. J., eds. *The Mind of the Child Who is Said To Be Sick*. Springfield, Ill.: C. C. Thomas, 1983.

Coupey, S., and Cohen, M. "Special Considerations for the Health Care of Adolescents with Chronic Illnesses." *Pediatric Clinics of North America* 31(1984):211–19.

Cowen, L.; Mok, J.; Corey, M.; et al. "Psychologic Adjustment of the Family with a Member Who Has Cystic Fibrosis." *Pediatrics* 77(May 1986): 745–53.

Daherthy, W., and Campbell, T. *Journal of Contemporary Families in Healthcare*. Sage Publications, 1988.

Darling, R. B. "Parent–Professional Interaction: The Roots of Misunderstanding." In Seligman, M., ed. *The Family with a Handicapped Child: Understanding and Treatment*. New York: Grune and Stratton, 1983.

Deasy-Spinetta, P., and Spinetta, J. "Educational Issues for Children with Cancer." *Candlelighters Quarterly Newsletter*. 13(Summer 1989):2–7.

Deeley, T. J. *Attitudes to Cancer*. Southhampton, England: Camelot Press Ltd., 1979.

Denholm, C. J., and Ferguson, R. V. "Strategies to Promote the Developmental Needs of Hospitalized Adolescents." *Children's Health Care*. 15(Winter 1987):183–87.

Dragone, M. A. "Perspectives of Chronically Ill Adolescents and Parents on Health Care Needs." *Pediatric Nursing* 16(Jan./Feb. 1990):45–50.

Dunkel-Schetter, C. "Social Support and Cancer: Findings Based on Patient Interviews and Their Implications." *Journal of Social Issues* 40(1984): 77–98.

Eiser, C. *The Psychology of Childhood Illness* New York: Springer-Verlag, 1985.

Eisert, D.; Kulka, L.; and Moore, K. "Facilitating Play in Hospitalized Handicapped Children: The Design of A Therapeutic Play Environment." *Children's Health Care* 16(Winter 1988):201–08.

Erikson, E. *Childhood and Society*. 2nd ed. New York: Norton, 1963.

Evans, M. "Learning to Lose Fear." *Nursing Times* 83(April 29, 1987):55–56.

Frantz, T. T. *When Your Child Has a Life-Threatening Illness*. Washington, D.C.: Association for the Care of Children's Health and The Candlelighters Foundation, 1988.

Friedman, S. B., and Hoekelman, R. A. *Behavioral Pediatrics: Psychosocial Aspects of Child Health Care*. New York: McGraw-Hill, 1980.

Gabriel, H. P., and Danilowicz, D. A. "Open-heart Surgery for Congenital Heart Disease: Minimizing Adverse Psychological Sequelae in Families Facing Major High-Risk Surgery." In Christ, A. E., and Flomenhaft, K., eds. *Psychosocial Family Interventions in Chronic Pediatric Illness*. New York: Plenum Press, 1982.

Garfunkel, J. M., and Evans, H. E., eds. American Academy of Pediatrics, Committee on Hospital Care. *Hospital Care of Children and Youth* (Elk Grove Village, Ill.: 1986).

Gerring, J., and McCarthy, L. *The Psychiatry of Handicapped Children and Adolescents: Managing Emotional and Behavioral Problems.* Boston: College-Hill Press, 1988.

Gibbons, M. B., and Boren, H. "Stress Reduction: A Spectrum of Strategies in Pediatric Oncology Nursing." *Nursing Clinics of North America* 20(March 1985):83–103.

Gilgoff, I. S., and Dietrich, S. L. "Neuromuscular Diseases." In Hobbs, P. R., and Perrin, J. M., eds. *Issues in the Care of Children with Chronic Illness.* San Francisco: Jossey-Bass. 1985.

Gipson, W. T.; Sivak, E. D.; and Gulledge, A. D. "Psychological Aspects of Ventilator Dependency." *Psychiatric Medicine* 5(1987):245–55.

Goldberger, J. "Issue-Specific Play with Infants and Toddlers in Hospitals: Rationale and Intervention." *Children's Health Care* 16(Winter 1988):134–41.

Gonsalves-Ebrahim, L., and Kotz, M. "The Psychological Impact of Ambulatory Peritoneal Dialysis on Adults and Children." *Psychiatric Medicine.* 5(1987):177–85.

Gottlieb, S., and Portnoy, S. "The Role of Play in a Pediatric Bone Marrow Transplantation Unit." *Children's Health Care: Journal of the Association for the Care of Children's Health.* 16(Winter 1988):177–81.

Greenberg, L. W.; Jewett, L. S.; Gluck, R. S., et al. "Giving Information for a Life-threatening Diagnosis." *American Journal of Diseases of Children* 138(July 1984): 649–53.

Greenwald, H. P. *Social Problems in Cancer Control.* Cambridge, Mass.: Ballinger Publishing Company, 1980.

Grossman, F. K. *Brothers and Sisters of Retarded Children.* Syracuse: Syracuse University Press, 1979.

Harvey, D., ed. *Parent–Infant Relationships.* Perinatal Practice Series, Vol. 4. New York: John Wiley and Sons, 1987.

Hedenkamp, E. A. "Humanizing the Intensive Care for Children." *Critical Care Quarterly.* 3(1980):63–73.

Hewett S.; Newson, J.; and Newson, E. *The Family and the Handicapped Child.* Chicago: Aldine Publishing Co., 1970.

Higby, Donald J., ed. *The Cancer Patient and Supportive Care: Medical, Surgical, and Human Issues.* Boston: Nijhoff Martinus Publishers, 1985.

Hobbs, N., and Perrin, J. M., eds. *Issues in the Care of Children With Chronic Illness.* San Francisco: Jossey-Bass, 1985.

Hobbs, N.; Perrin, J. M., and Ireys, H. T., eds. *Chronically Ill Children and Their Families.* San Francisco: Jossey-Bass, 1985.

Holaday, B. "Challenges of Rearing a Chronically Ill Child: Caring and Coping." *Nursing Clinics of North America* 19(1984):361–68.

Hollenbeck, A. R.; Susan, E. J.; Nannis, E. D.; et al. "Children with Serious Illness: Behavior Correlates of Separation and Isolation." *Child Psychiatry and Human Development* 2(1980): 3–11.

Horowitz, F. D. "Child Development for the Pediatrician." *Pediatric Clinics of North America.* 29(April 1982).

Hyman, R.; Feldman, H.; Levin, R.; and Malloy, G. "The Effects of Relaxation Training on Clinical Symptoms: A Meta-Analysis." *Nursing Research* 38(July–August 1989):216–20.

Isles, P. "Children and Cancer: Healthy Siblings' Perceptions During the Illness Experience." *Cancer Nursing* 2(1979):371–77.

Jamison, R. N.; Lewis, S.; and Burish, T. G. "Psychological Impact of Cancer on Adolescents: Self-Image, Locus of Control, Perception of Illness and Knowledge of Cancer." *Journal of Chronic Diseases* 39(1986): 609–17.

Kaufman, J., and Hardy-Ribakow, D."Home Care: A Model of a Comprehensive Approach for Technologically-Assisted Chronically Ill Children." *Journal of Pediatric Nursing* 2(August 1987):244–49.

Kazak, A. E.; Reber, M., and Snitzer, L. "Childhood Chronic Disease and Family Functioning: A Study of Phenylketonuria." *Pediatrics* 81(February 1988):224–30.

Kellerman, J., and Katz, E. B. "The Adolescent with Cancer: Theoretical, Clinical and Research Issues." *Journal of Pediatric Psychology* 2(1977): 127–31.

Kellerman, J.; Rigler, D.; Siegel, S.; et al. "Psychological Evaluation and Management of Pediatric Oncology Patients in Protected Environments." *Medical and Pediatric Oncology* 2(1976):353–60.

Kellerman J.; Zelter, L.; and Ellenberg, L.; et al. "Psychological Effects of Illness in Adolescence: Anxiety, Self-esteem and Perception of Control." *Journal of Pediatrics* 97(1980):126–31.

Knudson, A., and Natterson, J. "Participation of Parents in the Hospital Care of Their Fatally Ill Children." *Pediatrics* 26(1960):482.

Konrad, P. N., and Ertl, J. E. *Pediatric Oncology.* Medical Outline Series, Vol. 4. Garden City, New York: Medical Examination Publishing Co., Inc., 1978.

Koocher, G. P. "Psychosocial Issues During the Acute Treatment of Pediatric Cancer." *Cancer* 58(1986):468–72.

Koocher G. P.; O'Malley, J. E. Gogan, J. L. et al. "Psychological Adjustment Among Pediatric Cancer Survivors." *Journal of Child Psychologists and Psychiatrists.* 21(1980):163–173.

Kubler-Ross, E. *Aids: The Ultimate Challenge.* New York: Macmillan, 1987.

Langbaum, T. S., and Rosenstein, B. J. *The Johns Hopkins Hospital Cystic Fibrosis Clinic Patient Handbook.* 1985.

Lansky, S. B. "Management of Stressful Periods in Childhood Cancer." *Pediatric Clinics of North America* 32(1983):625–31.

Lansky, S. B. and Cairns, M. U. Psychiatric Syndromes in Pediatric Oncology Patients. *Psychiatric Medicine* 5(1987):405–17.

Leukemia Society of America. *Emotional Aspects of Childhood Leukemia: A Handbook for Parents.* New York, 1989.

Levensen, P. M.; Pfefferbaum, B. J.; Copeland, D. R. and Silberberg, Y.; "Information Preferences of Cancer Patients Ages 11–20 Years." *Journal of Adolescent Health Care* 3(1982):9–13.

Levin, D.; Morriss, F.; and Moore, G. C.; eds. A *Practical Guide to Pediatric Intensive Care.* St. Louis: C. V. Mosby Company, 1984.

Lynman, M. J. "The Parent Network in Pediatric Oncology: Supportive or Not?" *Cancer Nursing* 10(1987):207–16.

Mabe, P. A.; Riley, W. T.; and Treiber, F. A. "Cancer Knowledge and Acceptance of Children with Cancer." *Journal of School Health* 57(February 1987):59–63.

Mador, J., and Smith, D. "Psychosocial Adaptation of Adolescents with Cystic Fibrosis." *Journal of Adolescent Health Care* 10(1988):136–42.

Magrab, P. R. "Psychosocial Development of Chronically Ill Children." In Hobbs, M., and Perrin, J. M., eds. *Issues in the Care of Children with Chronic Illness.* San Francisco: Jossey Bass Publishers, 1985.

Mattson, A., and Gross, S. "Social and Behavioral Studies on Hemophiliac Children and Their Families." *Journal of Pediatrics* 68:(1966):952.

Maul-Mellot, S. K., and Adams, J. N. *Childhood Cancer: A Nursing Overview* Boston: Jones and Bartlett Publishers, 1987.

McCalla, J. L. "A Multidisciplinary Approach to Identification and Remedial Intervention for Adverse Late Effects of Cancer Therapy." *Nursing Clinics of North America* 20(March 1985):117–30.

McCollum, A. T. *Coping with Prolonged Health Impairment in Your Child.* Boston: Little, Brown & Co., 1975.

McElheny, J. E. "Parental Adaptation to a Child With Bronchopulmonary Dysplasia." *Journal of Pediatric Nursing* 4(October 1989):346–52.

McWhirter, W. R., and Marsel, J. P. *Pediatric Oncology: An Illustrated Introduction.* Sydney: Williams & Wilkens and Associates, 1987.

Menke, E. M. "The Impact of a Child's Chronic Illness on School-Aged Siblings." *Children's Health Care* 15(Winter 1987):132–140.

Michielutte, R., and Disker, R. A. "Children's Perceptions of Cancer in Comparison to Other Chronic Illnesses." *Journal of Chronic Diseases* 35(1982): 843–952.

Monaco, G. P. "Resources Available to the Family of the Child With Cancer." *Cancer* 58(1986):516–21.

Nathanson, M. N., and Monaco, G. P. "Meeting the Educational and Psychosocial Needs Produced By a Diagnosis of Pediatric/Adolescent Cancer." *Health Education Quarterly* 10(Supp.; 1984):67–75.

National Cancer Institute. *Services Available for People with Cancer: National and Regional Organizations.* July 1986.

National Institutes of Health. *Coping with Cancer: A Resource for the Health Professional.* Publication no. 82-2080 (1982).

National Institutes of Health. *Help Yourself: Tips for Teenagers with Cancer.* Publication no. 87-2211. (June 1987).

National Institutes of Health. *Taking Time: Support for People with Cancer and the People Who Care About Them.* Publication no. 87-2059. Reprinted November 1986.

National Institutes of Health. *Talking with Your Child About Cancer.* Publication no. 87-2761 (April 1982).

National Institutes of Health. *Talking with Your Child About Cancer.* Publication no. 87-2761 (April 1987).

National Institutes of Health. *When Someone in Your Family Has Cancer.* Publication no. 86-2685 (December 1985).

National Kidney Foundation. *A Note To Parents of Children with End-Stage Renal Disease.* Publication no. 08-56-83 (December 1983).

Offer, D.; Ostrov, E.; and Howard, K. I. *The Offer Self-Image Questionnaire for Adolescence: A Manual.* 3rd ed. Chicago: Michael Reese Hospital, 1982.

O'Connell, S. "Recreation therapy: Reducing the effects of isolation for the Patient in the Protected Environment." *Children's Health Care: Journal of the Association of Children's Health.* 12(1984):118–21.

Oremland, E. K. "Work Dynamics in Family Care of Hemophilic Children." *Social Sciences & Medicine.* 26(1988):467–75.

Orenstein, D. M. *Cystic Fibrosis: A Guide for Patient and Family*. New York: Raven Press, 1989.

Owen, S. V., and Froman, R. D. "Replacing Negatives with Positives." *Maternal Child Nursing*. 12(Nov.–Dec. 1987):42–47.

Pass, M. D., and Pass, C. M. "Anticipatory Guidance for Parents of Hospitalized Children." *Journal of Pediatric Nursing* 2(August 1987):250–58.

Pearlman, L., and Scott, K. *Raising the Handicapped Child*. Englewood Cliffs, N.J.: Prentice Hall, 1981.

Pearson, J. E. R.; Cataldo, M.; Tureman, A.; et al. "Pediatric Intensive Care Unit Patients: Effects of Play Intervention on Behavior." *Critical Care Medicine*. 8(1980):64–67.

Perrin, E. C., and Gerrity, P. S. "Development of Children with a Chronic Illness." *Pediatric Clinics of North America* 31(February 1984).

Perrin, E. C., and Gerrity, P. S. "There's a Demon in Your Belly: Children's Understanding of Illness," *Pediatrics* 67 (June 1981):841–49.

Perrin, J. M., and MacLean Jr., E. "Children with Chronic Illness: The Prevention of Dysfunction." *Pediatric Clinics of North America* 35(December 1988):1325–37.

Philips, H. C. *The Psychological Management of Chronic Pain: A Treatment Manual*. Springer Series on Behavior Therapy and Behavioral Medicine, Vol. 19. C. M. Franks, series ed. New York: Springer Publishing Company, 1988.

Pidgeon, V. "Compliance with Chronic Illness Regimens: School-Aged Children and Adolescents." *Journal of Pediatric Nursing* 4(February 1989): 36–47.

Pizzo, P. A., and Poplack, D. G., eds. *Principles and Practice of Pediatric Oncology*. Philadelphia: J. B. Lippincott Company, 1989.

Pochedly, C. ed. *Cancer Therapy in Children*. Thorofare, NJ.: Slack, 1983.

Pratt, L. *Family Structures and Effective Health Behaviors: The Energized Family*. Boston: Houghton Mifflin Company, 1976.

Prugh, D. G. *The Psychosocial Aspects of Pediatrics*. Philadelphia: Lea & Febiger, 1983.

Pruitt, D. B., and Strickland, M. "Psychological Factors Affecting Children's Response to Medical Procedures: A Guide for Clinicians." *Psychiatric Medicine*. 5(1987):199–208.

Reynolds, E. A., and Romenofsky, M. L. "The Emotional Impact of Trauma on Toddlers." *Maternal Child Nursing* 13(March–April 1988):106–09.

Riegel, B., and Ehrenreich, D. *Psychological Aspects of Critical Care Nursing*. Rockville, Md.: Aspen Publishers, Inc., 1989.

Ripple, R.; Biehler, R.; and Jaquish, G. *Human Development*. Boston: Houghton Mifflin Company, 1982.

Robinson, C. A. "Preschool Children's Conceptualization of Health and Illness." *Children's Health Care*. 16(Fall 1987):89–96.

Rosenbaum, P. L. "Prevention of Psychosocial Problems in Children with Chronic Illness." *Canadian Medical Association Journal* 139 (Aug. 15, 1988):293–95.

Ross, J. W.; Diserens, D.; and Turney, M. E. "Evaluation of a Symposium for Educators of Children with Cancer. "*Journal of Psychosocial Oncology* 7(1989):159–78.

Rubin, K. H.; Fein, G. G.; and Vandenberg, B. "Play." In Hetherington, E. M., ed. *Handbook of Child Psychology*, Vol. 4. *Socialization, Personality and Social Development*. New York: Wiley, 1983.

Russo, D. C., and Varni, J. W., eds. *Behavioral Pediatrics, Research and Practice*. New York: Plenum Press, 1982.

Ryan, N. M. "Stress-Coping Strategies Identified from School Age Children's Perspective." *Research in Nursing and Health* (1989):111–21.

Sabbeth, B. "Understanding the Impact of Chronic Childhood Illness on Families." *Pediatric Clinics of North America*. 31(February 1984):47–57.

Sahler, O. J. Z., and McArney, E. R. *The Child from Three to Eighteen*. St. Louis: C. V. Mosby Company, 1981.

Schowalter, J. E. "Psychological Reactions to Physical Illness and Hospitalization in Adolescence: A Survey." *Journal of the American Academy of Child Psychiatry* 16(1977):500–516.

Schwartz, S., and Miller, J. E. H. *The Language of Toys: Teaching Communication Skills to Special-Needs Children.* Kensington, Md.: Woodbine House, 1988.

Seligman, M., ed. "Siblings of Handicapped Persons." In M. Seligman, ed. *The Family with a Handicapped Child: Understanding and Treatment.* New York: Grune & Stratton, 1983.

Seligman, M. "Adaptation of Children to a Chronically Ill or Mentally Handicapped Sibling." *Canadian Medical Association Journal* 136(June 15, 1987) 1249–52.

Shandor Miles, M., and Carter, M. C. "Coping Strategies Used By Parents During Their Child's Hospitalization in an Intensive Care Unit." *Child Health Care.* 14(Summer 1985):14–21.

Shipman, A. *Parent Advocacy of the Chronically Ill Child.* Presented at the Second National Conference on Patient Education in Pediatrics, Washington, D.C.: November 2–4, 1989.

Siemon, M. "Siblings of the Chronically Ill or Disabled Child." *Nursing Clinics of North America* 31(June 1984):47–57.

Silbert, A. R.; Newburger, J. W.; and Fyler, D. C. "Marital Instability and Congential Heart Disease." *Pediatrics* 69(1982):747–50.

Silverman, M. M., and Katz, D. S. "Preventing Mental Health Problems." In R. E. K. Stein, ed. *Caring for Children with Chronic Illness: Issues and Strategies.* New York: Springer Publishing Company, 1989.

Simons, R. C., ed. *Understanding Human Behavior in Health and Illness.* 3rd ed. Baltimore, Md.: Williams & Wilkens, 1985.

Slaby, A. E., and Glicksman, A. S. *Adapting to Life-threatening Illness.* New York: Prager Publishers, 1985.

Slavin, L. A.; O'Malley, J. E.; and Koocher, G. P.; et al. "Communication of the Cancer Diagnosis to Pediatric Patients: Impact on Long-term Adjustment." *American Journal of Psychiatry* 139(1982):179–83.

Smith, G. "A Patient's View of Cystic Fibrosis." *Journal of Adolescent Health Care* 7(1986):134–38.

Steckel, S. B. *Patient Contracting*. Norwalk, Conn.: Appleton–Century–Crofts, 1982.

Steele, S. M. *Health Promotion of the Child with Long-term Illness*. 3rd ed. Norwalk, Conn.: Appleton–Century–Crofts, 1983.

Stein, R. E. K., ed. *Caring For Children With Chronic Illness: Issues and Strategies*. New York: Springer Publishing Company, 1989.

Stein, R., and Jessup, D. "A Noncategorical Approach to Chronic Childhood Illness." *Public Health Reports* 97(1982): 354–62.

Stepp-Gilbert, E. "Sensory Integration: A Reason for Infant Enrichment." *Issues in Comprehensive Nursing* 11(1988):319–31.

Steward, M. S. "Affective and Cognitive Impact of Illness on Children's Body Image." *Psychiatric Medicine* 5(1987):107–113.

Stoll, B. A., and Weisman, A. D. *Coping With Cancer Stress*. Boston: Martinus Nijhoff Publishers, 1986.

Thorne, S. E. and Robinson, C. A. "Health Care Relationships: The Chronic Illness Perspective." *Research in Nursing and Health*. 11(1988):292–300.

Triggs, E. G., and Perrin, E. C. "Listening Carefully. Improving Communication About Behavior and Development: Recognizing Parental Concerns." *Clinical Pediatrics* 28(April 1987): 185–93.

Vance, J. C.; Fazen, L. E.; Satterwhile, B.; et al. "Effects of Nephrotic Syndrome on the Family: A Controlled Study." *Pediatrics* 65(1980):948–955.

Van Eys, J., ed. *Children with Cancer: Mainstreaming and Reintegration*. New York: Spectrum Publications, 1982.

————, ed. *The Truly Cured Child: The New Challenge in Pediatric Care*. Baltimore: University Park Press, 1979.

Vessey, J. A.; Braithwaite, K. B.; and Wiedmann, M. "Teaching Children About their Internal Bodies." *Pediatric Nursing* 16(Jan.–Feb. 1990):29–33.

Waechler, E., Krulik, T.; Holaday, B.; and Martinson, I. M., eds. *The Child and Family Facing Life-Threatening Illness*. Philadelphia: J. B. Lippincott Company, 1987.

Waechter, E. H. "Children's Awareness of Fatal Illness." *American Journal of Nursing*. 71(June 1971):1168–72.

Wallace, M. H.; Reiter, P. B.; and Pendergrass, T. W. "Parents of Long-term Survivors of Childhood Cancer: A Preliminary Survey to Characterize Concerns and Needs." *Oncology Nursing Forum* 14(1987):39–43.

Walker, C. L. "Stress of Coping in Siblings of Childhood Cancer Patients." *Nursing Research*. 37(July–August 1988):208–12.

Walker, L.; Ford, M.; and Donald, W. "Cystic Fibrosis and Family Stress: Effects of Age and Severity of Illness." *Pediatrics* 79(February 1987):239–46.

Waters, B. G. H.; Ziegler, J. B.; Hampson, R.; et al. "The Psychological Consequences of Childhood Infection with Human Immunodeficiency Virus." *The Medical Journal of Australia* 149(August 15, 1988): 198–202.

Watson, M., and Greer, S., eds. *Psychosocial Issues in Malignant Disease*. New York: Pergamon Press, 1986.

Weitzman, M. "School and Peer Relations." *Pediatric Clinics of North America* 31(February 1984): 59–69.

Wentworth, E. H. *Listen to Your Heart: A Message to Parents of Handicapped Children*. Boston: Houghton Mifflin Co, 1974.

Wesolowksi, C. A. "Self-Contracts for Chronically Ill Children." *Maternal Child Nursing*. 13(February 1988): 20–23.

Whaley, L., and Wong, D. *Nursing Care of Infants and Children*. St. Louis: C. V. Mosby, 1983.

Whittey, C., and Roberton, N. R. C. "Parent–Infant Relationships in the Neonatal Intensive Care Unit." In Harvey, D., ed. *Parent–Infant Relationships*. Perinatal Practice Series, Vol. 4. New York: John Wiley & Sons, 1987.

Wilkinson, S. R. *The Child's World of Illness: The Development of Health and Illness Behavior*. Cambridge: Cambridge University Press. 1988.

SUGGESTIONS FOR FURTHER READING

American Cancer Society. *Back to School: A Handbook for Parents of Children with Cancer.* (#4662).

American Cancer Society. *Back to School: A Handbook for Teachers of Children with Cancer.* (#2640).

Berends, P. *Whole Child/Whole Parent: A Spiritual and Practical Guide to Parenthood.* New York: Harper & Row, 1983.

Bibace, R., and Walsh, M., eds. *Children's Conceptions of Health, Illness, and Bodily Functions.* San Francisco: Jossey-Bass, 1981.

Blum, R., ed. *Chronic Illness and Disabilities in Childhood and Adolescence.* Orlando, Fla.: Grune & Stratton, 1984.

Bopp, J., ed. *Activities for Children with Special Needs.* Washington, D.C.: Association for the Care of Children's Health, 1986.

Bowen, J. *When You Visit the ICU.* Washington, D.C.: Association for the Care of Children's Health, 1982. [Coloring book.]

Briggs, D. C. *Your Child's Self-Esteem: The Key to His Life.* New York: Doubleday, 1970.

Clarke, J. *Self-Esteem: A Family Affair.* New York: Harper & Row, 1980.

Cousins, N. *Anatomy of an Illness: As Perceived by the Patient.* New York: W. W. Norton, 1979.

Eisenburg, M. G.; Sutking, L. F.; and Jansen, M. A. *Chronic Illness and Disability Through the Life Span: Effects on Self and Family.* Vol. 4. New York: Springer Publishing, 1984.

Fassler, J. *Helping Children Cope: Mastering Stress Through Books and Stories.* New York: The Free Press, 1978.

Featherstone, H. *A Difference in the Family: Living with a Disabled Child.* New York: Penguin, 1980.

Franz, T. T. *When Your Child Has a Life-Threatening Illness.* Washington, D.C.: Association for the Care of Children's Health and the Candlelighters Foundation, 1988.

Good, J. D., and Reis, J. G. *A Special Kind of Parenting.* La Leche League, P. O. Box 1209, Franklin Park, Ill. 60131-8209.

Gortmaker, S. L., and Sappenfield, W. *Chronic Childhood Disorders: Prevalence and Impact.* Pediatric Clinics of North America, Volume 31, (1984): 3–18.

Hobbs, N. *The Futures of Children: Recommendations of the Project on Classification of Exceptional Children.* San Francisco: Jossey-Bass, 1975.

Hobbs, N., et al. *Chronically Ill Children in America: Background and Recommendations.* Nashville, Tenn.: Vanderbilt Institute for Public Policy Studies, 1983.

Kleinberg, S. *Educating the Chronically Ill Child.* Rockville, Md.: Aspen Systems, 1982.

Kuczen, B. *Childhood Stress: How to Raise a Healthier, Happier Child.* New York: Delta, 1987.

Massie, R. K. *The Constant Shadow: Reflections of the Life of a Chronically Ill Child.* In Hobbs and Perrin, 1985, 14–15.

McCollum, A. *The Chronically Ill Child: A Guide for Parents and Professionals.* Boston: Little, Brown & Co., 1981.

Miezio, P. M. *Parenting Children with Disabilities.* New York: Marcel Dekker, 1983.

Murphy, A. T. *Special Children, Special Parents: Personal Issues with Handicapped Children.* Englewood Cliffs, N.J.: Prentice-Hall, 1981.

Piaget, J. *The Child's Concept of the World.* New York: Humanities Press, 1951.

Pitzele, S. K. *We Are Not Alone: Learning to Live with Chronic Illness.* New York: Workman, 1986.

Plaut, T. F. *Children with Asthma: A Manual for Parents.* Amherst, Mass.: Pedipress, 1984.

Powell, T. H., and Ogle, P. A. *Brothers and Sisters: A Special Part of Exceptional Families.* Baltimore: Paul H. Brookes Publishing Co., 1985.

Rappaport, L. *Recipes for Fun: Play Activities for Young Children with Disabilities and Their Families.* Washington, D.C.: Let's Play to Grow, 1986.

Reisner, H., ed. *Children with Epilepsy: A Parent's Guide.* Kensington, Md.: Woodbine House, 1987.

Resnick, M., et al. *Minnesota Adolescent Health Survey.* Minneapolis: University of Minnesota, 1987.

Scheiber, B., and Moore, C. *Practical Advice for Parents: A Guide to Finding Help for Children with Handicaps.* 1981. Montgomery County Association for Retarded Citizens, 11600 Nebel St., Rockville, MD 20852.

Siminerio, L., and Betschart, J. *Children with Diabetes.* New York: American Diabetes Foundation, 1986.

Travis, G. *Chronic Illness in Children: Its Impact on Child and Family.* Stanford, Calif.: Stanford University Press, 1976.

INDEX